Medicine Cards

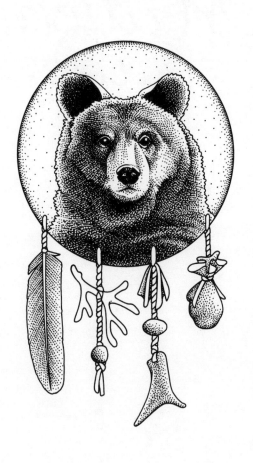

Medicine Cards

REVISED, EXPANDED EDITION

Jamie Sams & David Carson

Illustrations by Angela Werneke

ST. MARTIN'S PRESS ❧ NEW YORK

Card Concept: Jamie Sams & David Carson
Cover & Interior Design: Angela Werneke
Package & Card Background Art: James Finnell

ISBN 0-312-20491-4

10   9   8   7   6   5

It is with great love and respect that we dedicate this work to Grandmother Twylah for her lifetime of service to the teachings of the Wolf Clan and the children of Mother Earth. For *Ya-weh-node,* She Whose Voice Rides the Wind.

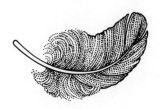

Contents

Contents————————9

Acknowledgments:

Thanks are due to Stephanie Hammer. Additionally, I would like to acknowledge my sweet medicine teachers, the women that passed to me the sacred teachings in trust: Opal, my mother; and my aunts, Ruby, Agnes, and Phoebe. May you all know that I have honored the Medicine and passed it on to those who could use it. I feel your hearts are smiling at me from the blue road of spirit and my heart is full. I am no longer "the invisible one."

David Carson

I would like to acknowledge my medicine teachers, the women and men who brought me through the void of Great Smoking Mirror. To Joaquin, my beautiful Mayan teacher; Grandfather Taquitz, who showed me unconditional love; Grandmother Twylah, who is my constant inspiration; and my two grandmothers, Olna and Verna, thank you for teaching me to touch the stars, to keep my heart open, and to walk my talk.

Jamie Sams

To our "sweet Nina" we send our love for holding the energy and typing her fingers to the bone. And to *all our relations*, we honor your life and light.

Introduction

In compiling the medicine that we have learned from the animal kingdom and our teachers throughout the years, we have discovered that these teachings need to be released in order to aid the mass consciousness. In the spirit of the Wolf Clan, we as teachers have therefore chosen to devise a method of divination to assist each soul to find its personal pathway through the medicine of animals.

The teachings vary from tribe to tribe, therefore we have used certain aspects of each animal's medicine to relay life lessons that apply to the human search for unity with *all our relations*. It is through nature that the teachings come, and it is to nature that we will all return. Each part of creation has a distinctive and valid place in the Medicine Wheel of all that is.

We are very fortunate to have been handed down these teachings from many elders in the Choctaw, Lakota, Seneca, Aztec, Yaqui, Cheyenne, Cherokee, Iroquois, and Mayan traditions. Due to the diverse teachings of these traditions, we have only scratched the surface of a deep understanding that is possible with this system of divination. Our purpose in creating this system is not to cover all the teachings on animal medicine that have ever been. Our intention, as shamans and healers, is to begin a process for many people who have never understood their connection to our Mother Earth and to all her creatures. We hope to open a new doorway of understanding for those who seek the Oneness of all life.

The visions that we have been given of this system are that it is a fun bridge which will aid in the understanding of what it means to "walk in balance on the Earth Mother." Our personal power animals have spoken to us through the Dream Lodge and have asked for our assistance in spreading the understanding that all life is sacred, and in sharing the lessons which they have to impart.

This system of divination and understanding has brought great medicine to our own lives and has been a very powerful and joy-filled journey in the making. It is a "give-away" from the four-leggeds, the creepy-crawlers, the finned ones, and winged-ones. May it enrich the lives of all of you whom it touches, and may all of you feel our love as you journey with us.

Four Winds,
Jamie Sams and David Carson

Dǎ nāho! Wi:yo:h!
(It is said! It is good!)

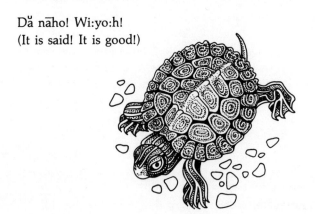

Animal Medicine

To understand the concept of medicine in the Native American way, one must redefine "medicine." The medicine referred to in this book is anything that improves one's connection to the Great Mystery and to all life. This would include the healing of body, mind, and of spirit. This medicine is also anything that brings personal power, strength, and understanding. It is the constant living of life in a way that brings healing to the Earth Mother and to all of our associates, family, friends, and fellow creatures. Native American medicine is an all-encompassing "way of life," for it involves walking on the Earth Mother in perfect harmony with the Universe.

Our fellow creatures, the animals, exhibit habit patterns that will relay these messages of healing to anyone astute enough to observe their lessons on how to live. The precious gifts of true medicine are free. Each lesson is based on one major idea or concept and, for the sake of simplicity, each animal has been assigned one of these lessons. In reality, each animal in creation has hundreds of lessons to impart, and all of those lessons are powers that can be called upon.

When you call upon the power of an animal, you are asking to be drawn into complete harmony with the strength of that creature's essence. Gaining understanding from these brothers and sisters of the animal kingdom is a healing process, and must be approached with humility and intuitiveness. Certain aspects of the lessons given by these brothers and sisters have been chosen to reflect the lessons each spirit needs to learn on the Good Red Road. These are the lessons of being human, being vulnerable, and seeking wholeness with all that is. They are a part of the pathway to power. The power lies in the wisdom and understanding of one's role in the Great Mystery, and in honoring every living thing as a teacher. The lessons taught are eternal and they are forever forthcoming. If the learning is over, so is the magic and the life.

This system of divination is one tiny aspect of the process of teaching a person how to be intuitive, how to seek the truths of nature, how to relate to the Great Mystery's creatures, and how to observe the obvious in the silence. This silence of the quiet mind is the sacred fertility of the receiving spirit. If you use this divination tool in silence, you will find a wondrous new world speaking to you through the ways of your fellow creatures.

It is possible to find animals that speak to you in a particular way — the way of power. These creatures may carry special medicine for you, and will call to you in the Dreamtime if you are to study them more closely. Your power ally is a certain species with which you have recognized an important connection. This species becomes your teacher, with whom you allow yourself to grow and learn. Nothing can replace the observation of these creatures in their natural habitats, for this connects you with the Earth, the animal, and the Great Mystery.

The spirit of the power ally may choose at times to enter the consciousness of one who has walked the Medicine Way for many years, and align itself to aid in healings. This is a part of the initiation process of Animal Medicine, and brings great power to the healer.

In learning to call on the medicine of any person, creature, or natural force, one must maintain an attitude of reverence and be willing to accept assistance. For instance, small native children know that if they are lost, they may call on the medicine of their parents. This brings to the child the strength of the parents, even though they are not physically present. The parents will feel the pull of the child's need, and oftentimes will be able to see psychically through the eyes of their child and determine its location. This is a kind of power that comes from the idea of unity, and of each being having within itself a part of all other beings. It is the law of oneness.

It is also possible to call upon the power or medicine of an animal when one is in need of specific talents. As all things in this universe have the same building block — the atom — it is relatively safe to assume that we all communicate through the common denominator of each atom, which is the creative force or Great Spirit that lives *within* the Great Mystery. It is the teaching of these truths that has brought native people to understanding, and it is these same truths that may open this door for you.

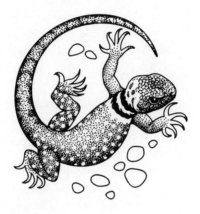

The Healing Powers of the Animal Medicines

In ancient times, an initiate, seeker, or person needing guidance would come before the elders. The elders were usually six in number and sat in the North. The elders were wise, not simply because they had led a long life, but because they knew the inner secrets. They understood the Wolf trails of the mind, experienced many powerful visions, and owned their powers as gifts.

Picture, if you can, a roaring Council fire and six elders sitting in the North under a new crescent Moon. The crescent Moon is drawn on the Earth in corn pollen. Three elder men sit on the left as you approach from the South, and three elder women sit on the right. In the darkness, the old ones are splashed in firelight. You sit in front of the second, or middle, man. His fierce, birdlike eyes hold you like a vise. He holds up a beaded medicine bag or pouch. It is covered in symbols and power designs and it is fringed on the bottom.

The middle man motions for you to reach inside. You do so. You pull out, perhaps, a Wolf tooth or Bear claw. He tells you to place it on the ground between the two of you, in a specific position. You do so. Then you take other items from the pouch and place them with the first item. Each position or direction has meaning and each object is a lesson or talent.

The middle woman looks at the objects you have selected and at the configurations you have placed them in. She begins speaking to you in a soothing voice. She seems to know all about you. She seems to reach inside to your very soul. She is a guide and a wise counselor. She is able to tell you if and how you have parted from your trail. She is able to tell you if some mischievous person or power has tricked you and how they have done so. She is able to advise you on any health problems you may have. She is able to guide your spiritual development. She causes you to look within yourself as never before, and you discover your harmony with all creation. She is able to give you advice on any question. When you leave the elders, you feel empowered and able to meet any situation. You feel complete.

The need for this type of guidance exists today. This is the function of the Medicine Cards. We are in an age that has severed itself from nature and magic. The Medicine Cards are a method for remedying that dissociation.

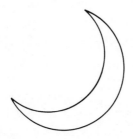

The Nine Totem Animals

Each and every person has nine power or totem animals that represent the medicine they carry in their Earth Walk. These animal or creature beings emulate each person's abilities, talents, and challenges.

For instance, if a person is connected to Wolf as a power animal, that person is a born teacher, pathfinder, innovator, and self-starter. This does not necessarily mean that the person has acknowledged those gifts and is using them to the fullest. It can mean that Wolf is there to bring that person to an understanding of the talents that need developing. If the person is ignoring those talents, you might say that Wolf would be appearing in the contrary.

As you come into this Earth Walk, there are seven directions surrounding your physical body. These directions are East, South, West, North, Above, Below, and Within. The direction called Within exists within you, but also surrounds you, since the entire universe is inside of your consciousness. You have a totem animal in each of the seven directions to teach you the lessons of these directions. To find these totem animals for yourself, spread the cards face down in front of you in an arc. Then get a piece of paper and begin by writing the direction East, for East is the "golden door" or entry point on the Medicine Shield. Write East, South, West, North, Above, Below, and Within on the left side of your paper. Quiet yourself, and ask in a reverent manner that the creature beings which are your silent guides and helpers guide your hand to their cards. The first card will be your animal of the East; the second card you pull will be your totem of the South; and so on for all seven directions. Write these animals down next to the directions on your piece of paper. These selections may surprise you, but they will be correct. By using this intuitive process, you, as the seeker, will connect with your proper guides. Once you have finished

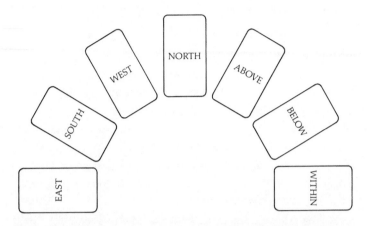

the selection of your seven animals for the seven directions, you should not do this process again. These are the creature beings that are your medicine.

The other two animals which make up your nine totems are the ones that are walking at each side of you at all times, and that may have been coming to you for years in dreams. If they have not come to you in dreams, they may be animals that you are drawn to but which have not appeared amongst the seven you selected. You may find that these last two creatures will appear for you at a later date. Or, when you read the qualities of the animals in this book, you may simply "connect" with the two that walk at your sides. However, the two that walk by your sides may not be in this text. They may be from any part of the animal kingdom on our Mother Earth. One of them could be a condor, a koala, a wolverine, or a chipmunk. To better understand the medicines of these animals, consult a book on their habits, and see how their characteristics apply to both humankind and yourself.

Your opinions of yourself cannot get in the way when you pick these cards, therefore you will tend to learn more about your true nature when you simply allow the animals to come to you.

SIGNIFICANCE OF THE NINE TOTEM ANIMALS

East: The animal in the East guides you to your greatest spiritual challenges and guards your path to illumination.

South: The animal in the South protects the child within and reminds you when to be humble and when to trust, so that innocence will be balanced in your personality.

West: The animal in the West leads you to your personal truth and inner answers. It also shows you the path to your goals.

North: The North animal gives wise counsel and reminds you when to speak and when to listen. It also reminds you to be grateful for every blessing every day.

Above: The Above animal teaches you how to honor the Great Star Nation, and reminds you that you came from the stars and to the stars you will return. This animal is also the guardian of the Dreamtime — for your personal access to the other dimensions.

Below: The Below animal teaches you about the inner Earth, and how to stay grounded and on the path.

Within: The Within animal teaches you how to find your heart's joy and how to be faithful to your personal truths. It is also the protector of your sacred space, the place that is yours alone and is never shared except by invitation.

Right Side: This animal protects your male side and teaches you that, no matter where you turn, it will be your Father-protector within. This animal also carries your courage and warrior spirit.

Left Side: This animal is the protector of your female side and teaches you that you must learn to receive abundance as well as to nurture yourself and others. The left-side animal is also your teacher about relationships and mothering.

The Medicine Wheel

All space is sacred space. Every inch of Mother Earth holds a specially energized connection to some living creature, and is therefore to be honored. The Medicine Wheel is a physical expression of this knowledge, and can be used to set up sacred ceremonial space. It is constructed by placing twelve large stones in a circle, similar to the face of a clock. The four largest stones are placed at the four cardinal directions. Begin by placing the stone in the South, the place of the child, where life begins. Then move to the West, to the North, and finally to the East. The Eastern stone is placed last because the space inside of the circle is filled by spirit entering through the Eastern door. The golden door to illumination is this Eastern door. When it is about to be closed, it is time to ask spirit to fill the space so that mutual honoring and love can occur. This is one of the traditional ways to build a Medicine Wheel.

The Medicine Wheel is used to gather together the energies of all the animals or creature beings, the Stone People, Mother Earth, Father Sky, Grandfather Sun, Grandmother Moon, the Sky World or Star Nation, the Subterraneans, the Standing People or trees, the Two Leggeds or humans, the Sky Brothers and Sisters, and the Thunder Beings. These we consider to be *all our relations* in the Native teachings.

Ceremony is a method for honoring and recognizing the connections to all life through the expression of gratitude in chants, dances, and rituals. It is always done with the guidance of Great Spirit and the Great Mystery.

The Medicine Wheel is a symbol for the wheel of life, which is forever evolving and bringing new lessons and truths to the walking of the path. The Earth Walk is based upon the understanding that each one of us must stand on every spoke of the great wheel of life many times, and that every direction is to be honored. Until you have walked in others' moccasins or stood on their spokes of the wheel, you will never truly know their hearts.

The Medicine Wheel teaches us that all lessons are equal, as are all talents and abilities. Every living creature will one day see and experience each spoke of the wheel and know those truths. The Medicine Wheel is a pathway to truth and peace and harmony. The circle is never ending, life without end.

In experiencing the Good Red Road, one learns the lessons of physical life, or of being human. This road runs South to North in the circle of the Medicine Wheel. After the graduation experience of death, one enters the Blue or Black Road that is the world of the grandfathers and grandmothers. In spirit, one will continue to learn by counseling those remaining on the Good Red Road. The Blue Road of spirit runs East to West.

The Medicine Wheel is life, afterlife, rebirth, and the honoring of each step along the way.

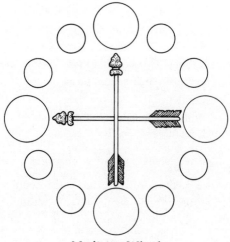

Medicine Wheel

The Medicine Shield

The Medicine Shield is an expression of the unique gift its maker wishes to impart about his or her current life journey. A Medicine Shield can speak of a new level in personal growth or it can illustrate the next mountain a person wishes to climb.

Traditionally, the shield a warrior carried spoke of the inner strengths he would use to help the tribe. The shield of a Native woman spoke of her gifts of nurturing and her talents in the areas of vision, healing, weaving, magic, singing, dancing, and beading. Shields spoke of their bearers' places in the tribal family and of the totems they carried.

By invoking recognition for the gifts of another, the Medicine Shields were a way to create harmony in the family, tribe, and nation. Shields spoke of the inner truths as well as the outer personalities of their makers. Each woman made her own shield. Each man would choose a brother who honored his own medicine to make his shield. This was to prevent the male ego from getting in the way of truth. Women were already connected to their intuitive sides and were more readily able to receive what their beading "voices" told them about their gifts. Women also understood the concept of sisterhood and left the role of protector to the men, while they took the role of Mothers of the Creative Force. Thus women made their own shields with humility and creativity.

To lie about your gifts was a great disgrace. To lie about anything, for that matter, could cause permanent exile from the tribe. Those who had lied and been exiled usually found jobs servicing white men as guides, or assisting the cavalry as forked-tongue interpreters. Shields that had lied were burned in a ceremony of great mourning, and the makers of these shields became invisible to the others of the tribe and nation.

Many times a shield would be made for the initiation of a project, and would contain the desired outcome. Other shields would be made to tell stories of a battle, a hunt, or a Vision Quest. When a special ceremony was to be celebrated, a shield would be made to depict the joy of the tribe and the spirits that would interact with the people. Shields were made as talismans for easy births, abundant harvests, or as signs of rites-of-passage into manhood or womanhood.

When a marriage was to take place, the shields of the bride and groom were placed opposite their respective owners in order to reveal the inner secrets of the partner's soul to the intended. After the bride and groom had jumped the fire together, the shields were hung on lances that crossed and joined as one on the door of the wedding lodge. These shields also went to the pole lodges with those who crossed over into the world of spirit. This was a sign of successful completion of the Earth Walk, and signalled the talents of the person crossing over to the grandfathers and grandmothers who had gone before.

A Sundance Shield is made as a symbol of the male dancer's desire to sacrifice the flesh of his body for world peace. This shield is a sign of the life patterns which that warrior is giving away within himself to promote both world peace and self-harmony. It speaks of his desire to come in humility, to dance the Sun in light, to seek the vision of what is needed, and to bear the pain of all our relations.

The secret shields of the women of the moon lodge speak of these women's talents and inner strengths that support their sisters. These shields are never shown to the outside world, since each one represents the sacred inner space of its maker. Each woman reveals her inner self to her sisters in complete trust, but never shows her total face to the outer world. This is to protect the creative force she carries in her womb-space, the force that follows the rhythms of the Earth and Moon.

Every shield carries medicine. Through its art and self-expression, each shield is the essence of a time and space that carries certain aspects of knowledge. All persons carry shields of the lessons they personally learned from the four directions on the Medicine Wheel. These lessons can be inclusive of their strengths and weaknesses, their talents and gifts, and their visions, purposes, and places in life. The totem of each direction can be expressed through a feather, a paw print, a symbol, or a piece of the totem animal's horn, tooth, bone, hide, fur, or fin.

Each shield is, for its maker, a reminder of his or her connection to life. In times of uncertainty, a Medicine Shield is a source of comfort, a source of protection from fear, and a reminder of the serenity of centered knowingness and connection. To balance the energy of uncertainty, the shield is meditated upon by its maker. As he or she enters the silence, questions of self-mystery are answered.

Medicine Shields represent signposts that guide our passage to wisdom and completion. It is the task of this Earth Walk to balance the shields of Self. In striving to be whole, we reflect the harmony, as well as the discord, of our many fragments.

Medicine Shields remind us of the fact that all things have their perfect time and place in life. Joys are balanced by tears, sacred silence by irreverent clowning, self-esteem by humility, giving by receiving, day by night, light by shadow, and wisdom by innocence. To walk in balance is to honor all acts of humanness in their proper times, and to find sacredness in them all.

Medicine Shields are the healing tools we give ourselves to soothe the spirit and empower the will. The truth needs no explanation, just reflection. This allows intuition to guide the heart so that humankind may celebrate more than it mourns.

The Medicine Card Spreads

The cards that come with the Medicine Cards system are numbered, and each card depicts on its face an animal inside a medicine shield. If the card is reversed, its number and animal will be upside down. Two lessons are therefore presented with each card: one for the right-side-up position and one for the reversed, or contrary, position.

It is always best to right all the cards before beginning. The cards may then be shuffled or mixed in any way you choose. After shuffling, place all the cards face down, so that you cannot see the drawings of the animals. Spread the cards on the table and choose one card for a daily meditation. Then, in silence, after reading the information about the card in the book, allow the animal to speak to you about what else it wants to teach you. You may also intuit how the lesson applies to your life situation, or to a particular challenge which you are facing.

THE PATHWAY SPREAD

Another method for using the cards is an ancient spread that comes from a Druidic system of divination. This spread gives you overall information about your pathway in life. The cards are laid out as illustrated.

This is how you would interpret the meaning of each card:
1) Your past
2) Your present
3) Your future
4) The pattern or set of life lessons that is moving through your life
5) The challenge you have conquered or the lesson just completed
6) What is working for you
7) What is working against you

By using this ancient Druidic spread, you are able to see

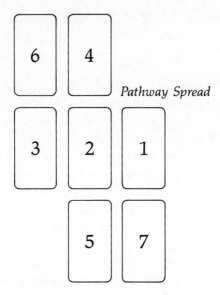

Pathway Spread

your present pathway as well as where you have been, where you are going, what is challenging you, and what you have completed.

THE MEDICINE WHEEL SPREAD

In the Medicine Wheel Spread, each of the four directions reveals certain things that you need to reflect upon in your personality. They also disclose how you are learning from yourself, from others, and from the animals. The card in the center is the Sacred Mountain or Sacred Tree position.

1) **The East card:** The card in this position reveals where your spiritual strength lies, and indicates the direction your spiritual path is taking. It can also reveal the major challenge to seeing clearly in your present situation.

2) **The South card:** The card in this position describes how its animal medicine is teaching the child within you, as your adultself walks through life. It is what you need to trust in yourself and what you need to nurture in your growing process.

3) **The West card:** The card in this position gives you the internal solution to your present life challenges. It indicates where your

goals need attention and how to reach the desired end.

4) **The North card:** The card in this position teaches you how you may spiritually apply and integrate the lessons of the other directions. The Animal Medicine of the card appearing in the North is the key to walking in wisdom, knowing the teacher within, and connecting to the higher-self's purpose and intention.

5) **The Sacred Mountain card:** The position of the Sacred Mountain asks you to look at the present. In this position you are standing, in a sense, at the crossroads of the spiritual and physical realities. This card will therefore indicate how your spiritual and physical realities have melded to produce the "you" of the present moment. Since all things evolve, tomorrow this "you" will have grown in understanding and your card may be different. In accepting this omen of who you are in the present, you may then see what needs changing or modifying, whether you are balanced or upset, and if you need to enter the silence for answers.

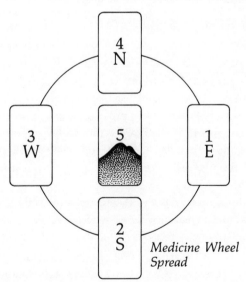

Medicine Wheel Spread

THE SUN LODGE SPREAD

This is another medicine wheel spread of the cards, but it determines how others see you. It is the spread of outward relationships, and in using it you are asking the medicine powers to tell you how another person perceives you. It is laid out in exactly the same manner as the previous spread, but with this difference: while doing the spread, you need to hold the image of the person you are asking about in your mind.

1) **The East card:** This card is an indication of how the person sees you spiritually.

2) **The South card:** This card is an indication of how the person sees you in relation to the material world.

3) **The West card:** This card is an indication of how the person is likely to interact with you in response to your deepest desires.

4) **The North card:** This card is an indication of how the person views you intellectually.

5) **The central card:** This card is an indication of the total view the person is likely to have of you. It suggests how the person will immediately respond to your presence.

THE MOON LODGE SPREAD *(Inward Tree for Centering)*

"There are more roots than branches," the old wise ones said.

This expression notes the importance of knowing what is beneath the surface. The Moon Lodge Spread is a mirror of your own personal unconscious. The world knows you outwardly, but only you can know the forces moving deep within yourself. The Moon Lodge Spread is therefore a tool to help you uncover that which is hidden. By using this spread, it is possible to rip away the veil of lies and self-deceptions you have been using to thwart your growth.

The Moon Lodge Spread is laid out in exactly the same manner as the previous medicine wheel spreads.

1) **The East card:** In the Moon Lodge Spread, this card is known as the Whirling Spirit Card. It is the key to unlocking your spiritual nature and to clearly seeing your spiritual talents and abilities.

2) **The South card:** This card is the new growth card or seed card. Look to this card for possible beginnings either in personal relationships or in how you relate to the environment. In the Moon Lodge Spread, this card may reveal your true feelings

about someone or something. It is the card that will show you your hidden emotion toward a person or thing.

3) **The West card:** This is the Dream-Within-the-Dream Card. It may lead you to your real purpose in life, so study it carefully. Is your dream or vision a product of your superficial ego, or are you being truly introspective and realizing the goals which your higher self is suggesting? It is here in the West that you impregnate yourself with your real life mission.

4) **The North card:** This card indicates the inner wisdom you may not have recognized in yourself. The North is the place of wisdom and knowing, therefore, if you are looking outside for answers, this card gently nudges you into following the animal's lead to find the same wisdom within yourself. Studying this card with the idea of knowing yourself will break any self-deception you may have.

5) **The central card:** This card indicates the integration point of all the directional medicines of your personal unconscious. It is the power shield of the True Self. This is the card of the circle of knowing the Within, the taproot of your personal consciousness. Know the True Self, the Within, and those without can never again deceive you.

THE BUTTERFLY SPREAD

This spread is used to determine the outcome of projects or group enterprises. Four cards are drawn and placed in the classic directional positions on the medicine wheel, i.e., East, South, West, and North. These cards will indicate the various phases your project or activity will move through toward its conclusion.

1) **The East card:** This card is known as the Egg Card or Egg Position. You should view this card as the nucleus or seed of your idea, project, or activity. Allow its medicine to interact with the concept of your enterprise. It will suggest the value of the inner core of your plan. Is it the medicine that is needed at this time or place?

2) **The South card:** This card is known as the Larva Card or Larva

Position. This card is about early doing. What needs to be done, and how will it be done, in the pragmatic world? Who will take responsibility for this work? Just as a butterfly egg first turns into a growing, struggling caterpillar, this is the medicine of the Larva Card. Will the energies be great enough to overcome the obstacles? The caterpillar sheds its skin many times during its growth. Will the many egos involved in your project or activity acquiesce (shed skin) in order to facilitate achievement?

3) **The West card:** This card is known as the Cocoon Card or Cocoon Position. It speaks of higher purpose. It is where the highest transformation takes place, much as when transformation happens inside the cocoon and a beautiful butterfly soon emerges. In viewing this card it is good to ask yourself why you have joined the activity or project you are considering. Was it to serve the Great Spirit and the tribe, or was it to serve yourself? If your activity or project was simply self serving, it will in all probability backfire on you. Not the self, but the family, the clan, the people, and the Great Spirit are to be served.

4) **The North card:** This card is known as the Butterfly Card or Butterfly Position. It is likely to tell you if the Great Spirit has

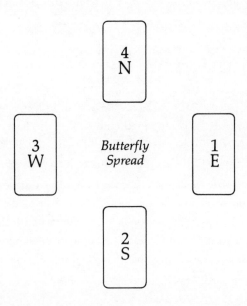

walked hand-in-hand with you and your group or project. Look to this card to tell you what sorts of rewards are to be gained. Will financial rewards be yours? It may seem odd to you to look to the North — the Spirit — for this answer. But as every medicine person will point out to you, *matter follows vision and spirit*. It is the law. This card is the place of manifestation.

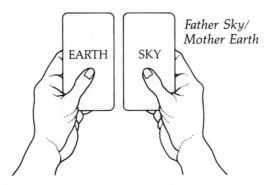

Father Sky/ Mother Earth

FATHER SKY/MOTHER EARTH SPREAD

This spread is a method for balancing yourself when times are hectic and you feel there is a need to rid yourself of confusion.

Every being has two sides to its personality: the female side or self, and the male side or self. Your male side is warrior energy: not war-like energy, but rather demonstrative energy. It is the side of you that has the courage to move forward, and the part of your being that is the protector of all you create. The male portion of you chooses to move forward into the world and seek adventure or to put ideas into action. It can be the father within who is always there to teach and console you. It can also be the medicine man within who knows how to heal you with his shamanistic ways. Father Sky relates to the right side of the body, which is ruled by the left brain, or analytical side of the mind. The Father Sky card is the present embodiment of these aspects of yourself.

The Mother Earth side of the body is the left side, the female side, which is ruled by the right brain, or intuitive side of the mind. The female receptive side of your nature knows how to allow the manifestation of life, and how to receive goodness through the process of allowing all things their time. It is the goddess energy, the anima, the mother within, the wise-woman, and the enchantress, as well as the little girl. The Mother Earth card is the nurturing side of your nature that houses the creative force. Within the Great Mystery all things exist. The ideas that will be reality and have material form are all seeds in the time/ space of the intuitive side of your nature. Female energy may be mysterious because it is constantly giving birth to new ideas and life forms; hence the changeability of woman. This card is your creative nature and your ability to receive those ideas from the Great Mystery.

To use this spread, merely pick one card with your right hand and one card with your left hand. Hold them in front of you and focus on the balance of your male-self (right) and your female-self (left). This process of observing the connection, or lack of connection, between your male and female sides will aid in balancing the energy between them. It is also possible, by placing these two cards side-by-side in front of you, or against your forehead if you are lying down, to balance your body's energy.

You may call upon the medicine of the creature beings, one at a time, to help balance the male and female sides within you. Be sure to enter the silence and allow the animals to speak to your heart. You may not hear words, but you may see pictures in your mind's eye. Then again, you may simply feel your energy moving and balancing itself. All of these sensations, as well as many more, are possible. All are correct. Whatever you feel, smell, sense, hear, or divine, is your way of understanding. You are developing your intuitive gifts, and these gifts will continue to grow and change the more you learn to trust your feelings and to *know*.

Editor's Note: Please remember to remove from your deck any blank shield cards that you have not filled in, prior to doing any of the *Medicine Card* spreads.

Contrary Cards

Whenever you find a contrary card in your spread, it indicates an imbalance in the medicine of that card. Its position in the spread will give you further information as to its meaning. If you wish to heal this condition but you do not readily understand how to right the upset balance and restore harmony, select another card and place it alongside the contrary card.

For example if you pull contrary Coyote, the most contrary card in the deck, and you are at a loss to understand how this card is instructing you, ask the cards to guide you by selecting another card. Place it next to the contrary card. Perhaps you pull contrary Antelope. This would signify that the answer lies in improper action. Or if you pull Skunk, this would imply that you are misreading cues about your reputation, and are perhaps reaching an erroneous conclusion about what others think of you.

After you practice using this method with each contrary card, you will be able to correctly interpret the proper energy to restore harmony to any indicated imbalance.

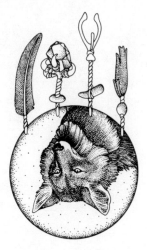

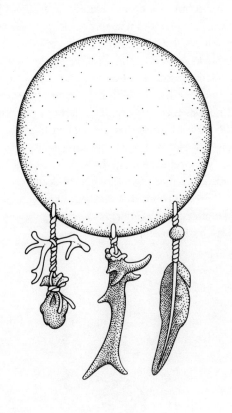

The Blank Shield Cards

Included in the Medicine Card deck are nine cards with blank shields on them. If you feel a close kinship with a certain animal which has not been included in the deck, such as an elephant, flamingo, trout, or mountain goat, we recommend that you write the name of that animal within the circle of one of these shields. This written name links the card with the animal's spirit through the principle of radionics, or vibration. Better still, paste a picture of your special animal within the boundaries of the shield's circle. You may then amend this card (or cards) to the deck, or carry it as a talisman on your person.

This same method may be used to create a Self shield, which can be amended to the deck. It may also be kept separately for use as the Sacred Mountain card or central card in a spread, to designate your energy. Use your artistic talent. Create a collage using pictures of the specific items you want in your life. Carry this card with you, preferably over or near your heart. Work with this Self card or collage card on your personal altar.

Use the nine blank cards for your nine totem animals. Place them in the nine directions or build a totem pole with them. Create shields for any member of your family. Create shields for power spots or meaningful places in your life. Perhaps you want to go on a vacation. Paste a picture of the Eiffel Tower inside the borders of a shield. Then call on the animal powers in the four directions and ask for their help in manifesting what you want. The same goes for a house or a car or anything else you may need. However, if you are working with the Medicine Cards to bring about your heart's desire, or to create another reality for yourself or someone else, never make a claim on a person who is married or on something that belongs to someone else. You may wish or work for something similar, but never for exactly the same thing that belongs to another. Do not break the laws of cause and effect. These cards are not meant as an aid to those who want to destroy another's creation.

The blank shields may also be used to create an Ally card. If you do shamanic work and have met your Ally on other levels of consciousness, you can create an Ally card for your personal use. An Ally is any particular alliance you have to the Creature-Beings, the Stone People, the Star Nation, the Finned Ones, the Creepy Crawlers, the Standing People (the trees), or any other living thing in nature. An Ally is your teacher and your guardian, a being that teaches the lessons of the physical and unseen worlds. Many Allies may come and go during your life.

As you can see, the blank shields may be used in a myriad of ways. If you work with a god or goddess energy, a card for this god or goddess may be created and used both in the deck and as a talisman. Use your creativity and talent. Meditate on the blank shield and see what comes to you. You may be surprised. The blank shield may act as the Great Smoking Mirror and reflect your inner desires, goals, dreams, power, or personality. Sometimes the emptiness of the blank shield will bring a vision of what lies below the surface of consciousness. Enjoy the journey of emptiness in this process, and the fulfillment will become pure creativity.

Medicine Cards

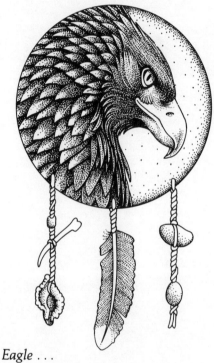

Eagle . . .
  Fly high,
    Touch Great Spirit.

Share your medicine,
  Touch me, honor me,
    So that I may know you too.

1
Eagle

Eagle medicine is the power of the Great Spirit, the connection to the Divine. It is the ability to live in the realm of spirit, and yet remain connected and balanced within the realm of Earth. Eagle soars, and is quick to observe expansiveness within the overall pattern of life. From the heights of the clouds, Eagle is close to the heavens where the Great Spirit dwells.

The feathers of Eagle are considered to be the most sacred of healing tools. They have been used for centuries by shamans to cleanse the auras of patients coming to them for healing. Within the belief systems of Native American tribes, Eagle represents a state of grace achieved through hard work, understanding, and a completion of the tests of initiation which result in the taking of one's personal power. It is only through the trial of experiencing the lows in life as well as the highs, and through the trial of trusting one's connection to the Great Spirit, that *the right* to use the essence of Eagle medicine is earned.

If you have pulled this symbol, Eagle is reminding you to take heart and gather your courage, for the universe is presenting you with an opportunity to soar above the mundane levels of your life. The power of recognizing this opportunity may come in the form of a spiritual test. In being astute, you may recognize the places within your soul, personality, emotions, or psyche that need bolstering or refinement. By looking at the overall tapestry, Eagle teaches you to broaden your sense of self beyond the horizon of what is presently visible.

In learning to fiercely attack your personal fear of the unknown, the wings of your soul will be supported by the ever-present breezes which are the breath of the Great Spirit.

Feed your body, but more importantly feed your soul. Within

the realm of Mother Earth and Father Sky, the dance that leads to flight involves the conquering of fear and the willingness to join in the adventure that you are co-creating with the Divine.

If Eagle has majestically soared into your cards, you are being put on notice to reconnect with the element of air. Air is of the mental plane, and in this instance it is of the higher mind. Wisdom comes in many strange and curious forms and is always related to the creative force of the Great Spirit.

If you have been walking in the shadows of former realities, Eagle brings illumination. Eagle teaches you to look higher and to touch Grandfather Sun with your heart, to love the shadow as well as the light. See the beauty in both, and you will take flight like the Eagle.

Eagle medicine is the gift we give ourselves to remind us of the freedom of the skies. Eagle asks you to give yourself permission to legalize freedom and to follow the joy your heart desires.

CONTRARY:

If you have pulled Eagle in the reverse, you have forgotten your power and connectedness to the Great Spirit. You may have failed to recognize the light that is always available for those who seek illumination. Heal your broken wings with love. Loving yourself as you are loved by the Great Spirit is the lesson which the contrary Eagle brings.

On some level, Eagle is telling you to seek higher ground on which to build your nest. The nest is the home of the heart and cannot remain in a swamp. If your nest is in a swamp, this may be connected to your belief that your wings are clipped by an impossibility in your present status.

Eagle's nest is high in the mountains, where the air is clean and the movement free. It may be your time for a Vision Quest so that you can commune with the Great Spirit. Fasting and praying will surely bring an answer. Seek lofty ideals, and illumination will be close at hand.

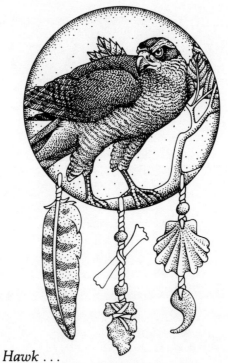

Hawk . . .
   Messenger of the sky,
      Circle my dreams and teach me
         The message as we fly.

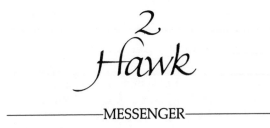

2
Hawk

---MESSENGER---

Hawk is akin to Mercury, the messenger of the gods. Hawk medicine teaches you to be observant, to look at your surroundings. Observe the obvious in everything that you do. Life is sending you signals.

Life *is* the initiation. If you have pulled the Hawk card, then right now a clue about the magic of life is being brought to you. This magic can imbue you with the power to overcome a currently stressful or difficult situation. The test is your ability to observe the nuances of power lurking nearby. Is power the talent you have and are not using? Are solutions always hard to find because you have lost the broader vision of Hawk? Or is the Great Spirit displaying a gift that you need only to receive? Have the colors of the morning inspired you to create? Or has the gloominess of a present situation left you earthbound, unable to hear the voice within the raindrops splashing on your window? Pay attention! You are only as powerful as your capacity to perceive, receive, and use your abilities.

What is called for here is an intuitive ability to discern the message carried within the cry of Hawk. The shrillness of Hawk's call pierces the state of unawareness, and asks you to seek the truth.

The Ancients recognized this magnificent bird of prey as a messenger bringing tidings to their Earth Walk, the Good Red Road, from the world of the grandfathers and grandmothers who lived before them. If Hawk were to magically cry, it was a sign to beware or be aware. This could mark the coming of a warring tribe, the birth of a child, or the celebration of counting coup. Hawk's cry signalled the need for the beholder to heighten awareness and receive a message.

Hawk medicine is a totem that is filled with responsibility, because Hawk people see the overall view. Hawk is not like Mouse, who sees everything through a magnifying glass. Hawk medicine people are aware of omens, messages from the spirit, and the color of the calling card you gave them three months ago. No detail slips by them unnoticed.

If Hawk has circled and landed in your card spread, you are to be aware of signals in your life — so notice and receive them. Hawk may be teaching you to grab an opportunity which is coming your way. On the other hand, Hawk may be bringing you the message that you should circle over your life, and examine it from a higher perspective. From this vantage point you may be able to discern the hazards which bar you from freedom of flight. Remember: Hawk has a keen eye and a bold heart, for Hawk flies close to the light of Grandfather Sun.

CONTRARY:

If you have drawn Hawk reversed, it may be because you have shut down your powers of observation on some level. If something in your life has become too painful to feel, too unbelievable to hear, or too dark to see, it is time to examine the point at which you chose to let yourself become emotionally involved, and to no longer be the observer. When you allow your emotions to override your perceptions, the message from Hawk cannot penetrate the chaos and confusion. At this point, you are asked to be mindful of the honest observer's neutral position, which allows the message to be intuitively and clearly understood, without emotion coloring its true meaning.

Emotional coloring is a tendency of Hawk medicine people when they are off-balance. Their emotions cloud their vision and lead to a crash landing. The ego can clip the wings and leave Hawk grounded. Also, if Hawk believes that those who cannot fly the same way he/she does have weaker perceptions, then the winged messenger has not understood his or her own medicine.

Freedom of flight is a privilege, and being a messenger is an honor. The responsibility for delivery of the message is up to

you. Take your flight and forget about interpreting the omen
your own way. Let the receiver decide what the message means.
After all, unless it was sent specifically for you, you would be
tampering.

Hawk in the contrary position teaches you:

1) To open up to the powers of observation

2) Not to tell others how to think or behave

3) To take care of your own emotional baggage before you begin
receiving omens, visions, or messages

4) To remember that all gifts are equal in the eyes of the
Great Spirit.

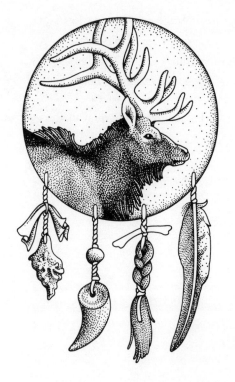

Elk . . .
   Your antlers reach for the Sun.

Show me that strength
            and stamina are one.

3
Elk

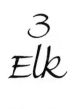

————————STAMINA————————

Elk wandered through the forest looking for a partner. The mating season was in full swing, and the bucks that usually traveled with the other males had dispersed to find mates for the season. As Elk bellowed his mating call through the forest, his bugling alerted Mountain Lion that a feast could be in the making.

Mountain Lion circled Elk, getting closer to his prey moment by moment. Elk sensed the impending danger when the forest grew suddenly silent. He broke for the high country when he spotted his pursuer, but Mountain Lion was far behind. As Elk made a running leap for the timberline, Mountain Lion gained on him, but Elk continued to run onward, displaying tremendous stamina. Finally Mountain Lion gave up, having spent his energy in spurts as he tried to jump over boulders to reach Elk. Elk paced himself, making headway as he climbed skyward toward the high country. Elk had no other defense except his ability to go the distance, setting a pace that allowed him to utilize his stamina and energy to the fullest.

Elk medicine teaches that pacing yourself will increase your stamina. Elk medicine people may not be the first ones to arrive at a goal, but they always arrive without getting burned out. If you have taken on too much recently, it might be a good idea to look at how you plan to finish what you have started without ending up in the hospital.

Elk have a curious kind of warrior energy because, except at mating time, they honor the company of their own gender. They can call on the medicine of brotherhood or sisterhood. In discovering the strength which is gained from loving the gender that is your own, you will feel the comradeship that arises from similarity of experience. This is a special medicine that allows the friendship of others of your same sex to overcome potential competition or jealousy.

If you have picked Elk medicine, you may be telling yourself to seek the company of your own gender for awhile. You may need a support group to realign yourself with the stamina of the warrior/warrioress energy that you are a part of. This communication with others of your own sex allows you to air your feelings in safety and to get feedback from others who have had the same experiences. You may need a new sense of community — communication in unity.

Elk could also be telling you to look at how you are holding up physically to the stresses in your life, and to pace yourself so that you maintain an equilibrium of energy over the distance you plan to cover. Vitamins or high-energy foods may be one solution, along with some personal quiet time for replenishment.

CONTRARY:

If Elk has appeared in the reverse position, you may be stretching the rubber band to the breaking point. Be careful of undue stress levels, or you might just create an illness to force you to take a break.

On another level, you may not be honoring your desire for companionship with the opposite sex, and you may have forgotten the excitement of mating season. If this is the case, you may find that your best option is to invite friends of the opposite sex for dinner or an afternoon outing. This is not to say that you would be sexually interested in these friends; it is merely suggesting that the exchange of opposite energies could be rewarding.

If you are in a relationship, it may be that the honeymoon is waning and that you need to stir up some excitement. Persistently creating a "change of pace" is the kind of stamina needed for any relationship to last.

In all cases, Elk is telling you to look at how you choose to create your present pathway, and how you intend to perpetuate it to reach your goal. Your best weapon is the same as Elk's:

to stop when you need to, to persist when you need to, and to allow room for change and exchange of energies.

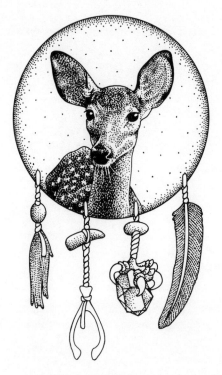

Deer . . . so gentle
  and loving you are.

The flower of kindness,
  an embrace from afar.

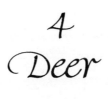

4
Deer

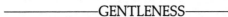
—————————GENTLENESS—————————

One day Fawn heard Great Spirit calling to her from the top of Sacred Mountain. Fawn immediately started up the trail. She didn't know that a horrible demon guarded the way to Great Spirit's lodge. The demon was trying to keep all the beings of creation from connecting with Great Spirit. He wanted all of Great Spirit's creatures to feel that Great Spirit didn't want to be disturbed. This would make the demon feel powerful, and capable of causing them to fear him.

Fawn was not at all frightened when she came upon the demon. This was curious, as the demon was the archetype of all the ugly monsters that have ever been. The demon breathed fire and smoke and made disgusting sounds to frighten Fawn. Any normal creature would have fled or died on the spot from fright.

Fawn, however, said gently to the demon, "Please let me pass. I'm on the way to see Great Spirit."

Fawn's eyes were filled with love and compassion for this oversized bully of a demon. The demon was astounded by Fawn's lack of fear. No matter how he tried, he could not frighten Fawn, because her love had penetrated his hardened, ugly heart.

Much to the demon's dismay, his rock-hard heart began to melt, and his body shrank to the size of a walnut. Fawn's persistent love and gentleness had caused the meltdown of the demon. Due to this gentleness and caring that Fawn embodied, the pathway is now clear for all of Great Spirit's children to reach Sacred Mountain without having to feel the demons of fear blocking their way.

Deer teaches us to use the power of gentleness to touch the hearts and minds of wounded beings who are trying to keep us from Sacred Mountain. Like the dappling of Fawn's coat, both the light and the dark may be loved to create gentleness and safety for those who are seeking peace.

If Deer has gently nudged its way into your cards today, you are being asked to find the gentleness of spirit that heals all wounds. Stop pushing so hard to get others to change, and love them as they are. Apply gentleness to your present situation and become like the summer breeze: warm and caring. This is your tool for solving the present dilemma you are facing. If you use it, you will connect with Sacred Mountain, your centering place of serenity, and Great Spirit will guide you.

CONTRARY:

Deer in the contrary position indicates that you are courting your fear by fighting the internal demons of negative ideas. This is a clue to you that force is not always the best method. You may not be willing to love yourself enough to feel your fears and let them go. You may be projecting your fears on others. It may also be others whom you fear, reminding you of a time when you reacted to life in much the same manner. At any rate, love is the key. The only true balance to power is the love and compassion of Deer. Be willing to find things to love about yourself and others, and your demons will melt away. Your fears cannot exist in the same place that love and gentleness abide.

Remember, Fawn can teach you many lessons about unconditional love. In its true application, unconditional love means that no strings are attached. The gentleness of Fawn is the heart-space of Great Spirit which embodies His/Her love for us all.

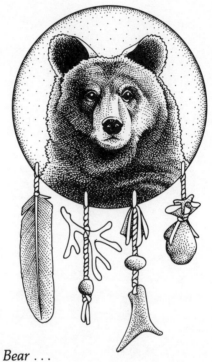

Bear . . .
    Invite me
        Into the cave
            Where silence surrounds

    The answers you gave.

5
Bear

The strength of Bear medicine is the power of introspection. It lies in the West on the great medicine wheel of life. Bear seeks honey, or the sweetness of truth, within the hollow of an old tree. In the winter, when the Ice Queen reigns and the face of death is upon the Earth, Bear enters the womb-cave to hibernate, to digest the year's experience. It is said that our goals reside in the West also. To accomplish the goals and dreams that we carry, the art of introspection is necessary.

To become like Bear and enter the safety of the womb-cave, we must attune ourselves to the energies of the Eternal Mother, and receive nourishment from the placenta of the Great Void. The Great Void is the place where all solutions and answers live in harmony with the questions that fill our realities. If we choose to believe that there are many questions to life, we must also believe that the answers to these questions reside within us. Each and every being has the capacity to quiet the mind, enter the silence, and *know*.

Many tribes have called this space of inner-knowing the Dream Lodge, where the death of the illusion of physical reality overlays the expansiveness of eternity. It is in the Dream Lodge that our ancestors sit in Council and advise us regarding alternative pathways that lead to our goals. This is the power of Bear.

The female receptive energy that for centuries has allowed visionaries, mystics, and shamans to prophesy is contained in this very special Bear energy. In India, the cave symbolizes the cave of Brahma. Brahma's cave is considered to be the pineal gland that sits in the center of the four lobes of the brain.

If one were to imagine an overview of the head, the top of

it would be a circle. The South would be the forehead, the North the back of the skull, the West would be the right brain, and the East the left brain.

Bear is in the West, the intuitive side, the right brain. To hibernate, Bear travels to the cave, which is the center of the four lobes where the pineal gland resides. In the cave, Bear seeks answers while he/she is dreaming or hibernating. Bear is then reborn in the spring, like the opening of spring flowers.

For eons, all seekers of the Dreamtime and of visions have walked the path of silence, calming the internal chatter, reaching the place of rites of passage — the channel or pineal gland. From the cave of Bear, you find the pathway to the Dream Lodge and the other levels of imagination or consciousness. In choosing Bear, the power of knowing has invited you to enter the silence and become acquainted with the Dream Lodge, so that your goals may become concrete realities. This is the strength of Bear.

CONTRARY:

If you have drawn Bear reversed, your internal dialogue may have confused your perception of your true goals. In seeking answers or advice from others, you may have placed your own feelings and knowing aside. The time has come to regain your authority, for no one knows better than yourself what is proper and timely for your evolution. Reclaim the power of knowing. Find joy in the silence and richness of the Mother's womb. Allow the thoughts of confusion to be laid to rest as clarity emerges from the West, nurturing your dreams as the Earth Mother nourishes us all.

Bear in the contrary position is teaching you that only through being your own advisor can you attain your true goals. Anything less than the doing of that which gives you the most joy is denial. To achieve happiness you must know yourself. To know yourself is to know your body, your mind, and your spirit. Use your strengths to overcome your weaknesses and know that both are necessary in your evolution.

Journey with Bear to the quietness of your cave and hibernate in silence. Dream your dreams and own them. Then in strength you will be ready to discover the honey waiting in the Tree of Life.

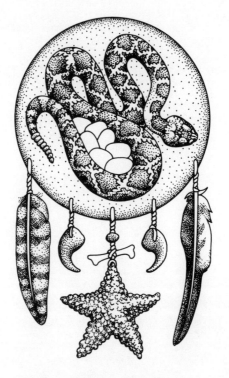

Snake . . . come crawling,
There's fire in your eyes.
Bite me, excite me,
I'll learn to realize,

The poison transmuted,
Brings eternal flame.
Open me to heaven,
To heal me again.

6
Snake

---TRANSMUTATION---

Snake medicine people are very rare. Their initiation involves experiencing and living through multiple snake bites, which allows them to transmute all poisons, be they mental, physical, spiritual, or emotional. The power of snake medicine is the power of creation, for it embodies sexuality, psychic energy, alchemy, reproduction, and ascension (or immortality).

The transmutation of the life-death-rebirth cycle is exemplified by the shedding of Snake's skin. It is the energy of wholeness, cosmic consciousness, and the ability to experience anything willingly and without resistance. It is the knowledge that all things are equal in creation, and that those things which might be experienced as poison can be eaten, ingested, integrated, and transmuted if one has the proper state of mind. Thoth, the Atlantean who later returned as Hermes and was the father of alchemy, used the symbology of two snakes intertwining around a sword to represent healing. Complete understanding and acceptance of the male and female within each organism creates a melding of the two into one, thereby producing divine energy.

This medicine teaches you on a personal level that you are a universal being. Through accepting all aspects of your life, you can bring about the transmutation of the fire medicine. This fire energy, when functioning on the material plane, creates passion, desire, procreation, and physical vitality. On the emotional plane, it becomes ambition, creation, resolution, and dreams. On the mental plane it becomes intellect, power, charisma, and leadership. When this Snake energy reaches the spiritual plane, it becomes wisdom, understanding, wholeness, and connection to the Great Spirit. If you have chosen this symbol, there is a need within you to transmute some thought, action, or desire so that wholeness may be achieved. This is heavy magic, but remember, magic is no more than a change in consciousness. Become the magician or the enchantress: transmute the energy and accept the power of the fire.

CONTRARY:

If you have drawn this symbol in the reverse, you may have chosen to mask your ability to change. Look at the idea that you may fear changing your present state of affairs because this may entail a short passage into discomfort. Does this discomfort keep you from assuming the viewpoint of the magician within? Is the old pattern safe, reliable, and a rut? In order to glide beyond that place which has become safe but nonproductive, become Snake. Release the outer skin of your present identity. Move through the dreamlike illlusion that has insisted on static continuity, and find a new rhythm as your body glides across the sands of consciousness, like a river winding its way toward the great waters of the sea. Immerse yourself in that water, and know that the single droplet which you represent is being accepted by the whole.

Feel Snake's rhythm and you will dance freely, incorporating those transmuting forces of the universe as a part of your sensual dance of power.

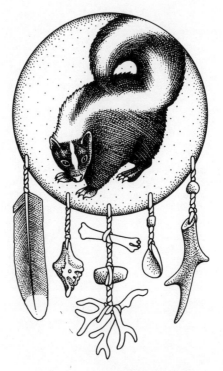

Skunk . . . tell me the story,
So I will know it well,
Of how to attract,
And how to repel.

7
Skunk

---REPUTATION---

Skunk medicine! Go ahead and laugh. This furry little animal has a reputation that contains a great deal of power. Due to its distinctive behavior, humans give this tiny, smelly creature a wide berth. The key word here is *respect*.

Unlike other predatory animals, Skunk does not threaten your life but threatens your senses. You know this to be true if you have ever been in the vicinity of its spray. In observing the habit patterns of Skunk, it is easy to notice the playfulness and nonchalance of its natural behavior. The "I-dare-you" attitude of this four-legged creature commands you, as the observer, to respect its space by mere reputation alone.

Skunk is teaching you that by walking your talk and by respecting yourself, you will create a position of strength and honored reputation. The carriage of your body relates to others what you believe about yourself. There is no need to bully, aggravate, torment, or overpower other beings when your sense of "self" is intact. As with Skunk, the resonant field of energy around your body is relayed through the senses. Self-esteem permeates the body's energy, and is instantly recognized on an extrasensory level by others.

Learn to assert, without ego, what you are. Respect follows. Your self-respectful attitude will repel those who are not of like mind, and yet will attract those who choose the same pathway. As the odor of Skunk attracts others of its kind, it repels those who will not respect its space.

Skunk medicine people have the ability to attract others, and they are very charismatic. At the same time, the other side of their natural power is to repel those who seek to take energy from them without recycling the gifts they have taken.

Skunk medicine people also know how to use the energy flows that will attract a lover. Some people call this sexual magic, as it is akin to the musk scent that animals excrete to attract a mate. It can be dangerous to leak sexual energy if you are not looking for a mate. It puts you into a games condition that may feed your ego but not how others feel about you. If you are attracting others who have an interest in you, you are in a sense saying, "I'm available." This can cause hard feelings when the truth comes out. It also leaks energy that you could have used in a more constructive way.

In Skunk medicine, it is good to learn how to handle energy flows. Modern psychologists call this body language. In tribal teachings, this is your personal medicine which you are showing to others. Use your medicine well, and know that you are known by your reputation. How you use your energy will attract either honor or disgrace. You may want to examine what energy you are putting out that creates your present situation.

If you have chosen this symbol, you are being asked to notice the kinds of people who are attracted to you. If they emulate favorable characteristics, have enough self-esteem to recognize those characteristics within yourself. Walk tall and be proud of the accomplishments you have made. Bear in mind that what you believe about yourself is your ultimate protection. Project self-respect!

CONTRARY:

Skunk medicine operating through the contrary or reversed position indicates that your self-esteem may seem to others as if you are putting on airs. Observe whether or not you are repelling others in your vicinity because of envy, jealousy, or a projection of *their* low self-esteem. Examine your feelings. Be truthful with yourself. Right the situation by assuming the attitude of Skunk: nonchalance. In assuming nonchalance, you are neutralizing the effect of leaking energy.

In leaking vital energy, you may be stinking up your environment. This is similar to dumping all of your woes on anyone who will listen. If you are doing this, it may be time to shut your mouth and go within. You may also be leaking sexual energy and repulsing the object of your interest. That person may be too shy to tell you to lay off. Look deeply at your self-image and how others are reacting to it.

To balance the causes and effects of your actions and energy flows, you must decide whether or not you need to spray in the direction of others to repel their envy, greed, jealousy, or over-amorous tendencies. On the other hand, you need to always maintain your "right to be." Self-respect is the key to all of these situations, whereas ego is merely what you believe yourself to be.

Skunk says, "If your ego is not your amigo, you know it stinks!"

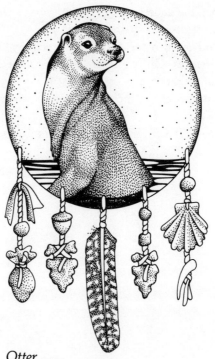

Otter . . .
    So playful!
        Coquettes by the stream.

The medicine of woman,
    The Realized Dream.

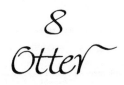

8
Otter

---WOMAN MEDICINE---

The medicine held by Otter is a set of lessons in female energy. This applies to both men and women, as all of us have female sides. The Otter's hide is very often used to make medicine bags for powerful women because it represents balanced female energy.

Otter is very caring of its young and will play for hours, performing all types of acrobatics. It lives on land, but always has its home near water. The elements of Earth and Water are the female elements. At home in both of these elements, Otter is the personification of femininity: long, sleek, and graceful, Otter is the true coquette of the animal world.

Otter is always on the move and is very curious. Unlike other animals, Otter will not start a fight unless it is attacked first. This joyful little creature is adventuresome and assumes that all other creatures are friendly — until proven otherwise.

These character traits are the beauty of a balanced female side, the side of ourselves that creates a space for others to enter our lives without preconceptions or suspicions. Otter teaches us that balanced female energy is not jealous or catty. It is sisterhood, content to enjoy and share the good fortune of others. Anchored in the understanding that *all* accomplishments are worthwhile for the whole tribe, Otter people express joy for others.

Long ago, in tribal law, if a woman were widowed, her sister would offer her own husband to the widow as a lover to keep her from drying up and not using her creative urges. This is Otter medicine, too. Envy, or the fear of being replaced, has no space in Otter's balanced understanding of sharing goodness.

Woman energy without games or control is a beautiful

experience. It is the freeness of love without jealousy. It is the joy of loving other people's children and their accomplishments as much as you love your own.

It may be time to examine your feelings about sharing the bounty of your life with others. Otter may be saying that the finer qualities of woman need to be striven for in both men and women so that a unity of spirit can be achieved. This would involve the destruction of jealousy and of all the acts of anger which stem from that fear. It would mean keeping a Hawk-eye on your ego and maintaining total trust. It would mean a world full of people coming together to honor the right of each person to *be*.

If you have drawn this symbol, Otter may be telling you to become the playful child and to simply allow things to unfold in your life. It may be time to stop your addiction to worrying. Otter also teaches the importance of not hanging onto material things that would bind you or become a burden. In looking at how you can learn from Otter's habits, you might look at the joyousness of the receptive side of your nature. Have you given yourself a gift recently? Have you received any messages in your meditations? Become Otter and move gently into the river of life. Flow with the waters of the Universe . . . this is the way of balanced female-receptive energy. Honor it! In doing so, you will discover the power of woman.

CONTRARY:

If the Otter card appears reversed, you may be running from one idea to another without focus. This could also imply that you have forgotten how to receive, and are blocking a gift from the Universe with your male side. If this is the case, you may be embarrassed to receive compliments, to have someone hug you, or to allow your genuine personality to come out. Fear of being rejected is the contrary message of Otter. Drop the seriousness on all levels and play at life so that the fear rolls off your back. Realize that the *only* flow is the flow of love from the Great Spirit to you, from you to others, and from others back to you.

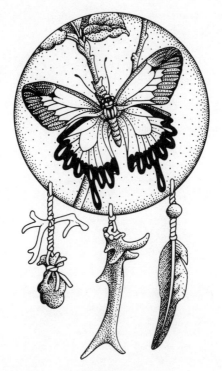

Butterfly . . . that flutters
  In the morning light,
    You have known many forms,
      Before you e'er took flight.

9
Butterfly

---TRANSFORMATION---

The power that Butterfly brings to us is akin to the air. It is the mind, and the ability to know the mind or to change it. It is the art of transformation.

To use Butterfly medicine, you must astutely observe your position in the cycle of self-transformation. Like Butterfly, you are always at a certain station in your life activities. You may be at the egg stage, which is the beginning of all things. This is the stage at which an idea is born, but has not yet become a reality. The larva stage is the point at which you decide to create the idea in the physical world. The cocoon stage involves "going within": doing or developing your project, idea, or aspect of personality. The final stage of transformation is the leaving of the chrysalis and birth. This last step involves sharing the colors and joy of your creation with the world.

If you look closely at what Butterfly is trying to teach, you will realize that it is the never-ending cycle of self-transformation. The way to discern where you are in this cycle is to ask yourself:

1) Is this the egg stage: Is it just a thought or idea?

2) Is this the larva stage: Do I need to make a decision?

3) Is this the cocoon stage: Am I developing and doing something to make my idea a reality?

4) Is this the birth stage: Am I sharing my completed idea?

By asking yourself these questions, you will discover how Butterfly is relating to you at this moment. When you understand where you are, the symbol can teach you what to do next to continue in the cycle of self-transformation. If you have found the position through which you are cycling, you will see the creativity of Butterfly.

Using the air, or mental powers, of this medicine is done with ease. As an example, if you have been feeling exhausted and have asked how to heal your fatigue, take notice of the colors you have been drawn to recently. Does your body feel better in green? Could this mean that you need to eat more green vegetables? This type of thinking is an inspiration from Butterfly medicine.

Butterfly can give clarity to your mental process, help you organize the project you are undertaking, and assist you in finding the next step for your personal life or career. The main message to be obtained from drawing this symbol is that you are ready to undergo some type of transformation. To discern what your next move is, use the Butterfly Spread.

CONTRARY:

If you have drawn Butterfly reversed, your lesson is a simple one. There is a need for change in your life that you are not recognizing. This could be a possible need for freedom, for a vacation, or for a new job. You may believe that change is too difficult, and you may rule it out to preserve the comfort of old habits. But in ruling out any possibility of change, you are saying that the courage of Butterfly has been lost. Why does Butterfly represent courage? Because there is a totally different world outside the cocoon, where the known realities of the chrysalis are no longer applicable. This new world demands that you use your newfound wings — and fly!

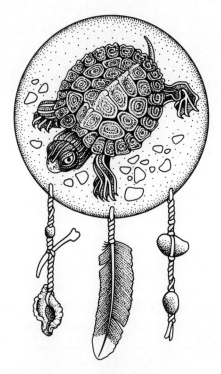

Turtle ... Great Mother,
Feed my spirit,
    Clothe my heart,

That I may serve you too.

10
Turtle

In Native American teachings, Turtle is the oldest symbol
for planet Earth. It is the personification of goddess energy, and
the eternal Mother from which our lives evolve. We are born of
the womb of Earth, and to her soil our bodies will return. In
honoring the Earth, we are asked by Turtle to be mindful of the
cycle of give and take, to give back to the Mother as she has
given to us.

Turtle has a shell which is similar to the protection that Earth
has employed for centuries as her body has been defiled. Mother
Earth's protection has come in the form of Earth changes, new
plant growth, the creation of new land masses by volcanoes,
and climate alterations. Like Turtle, you also have shields that
protect you from hurt, envy, jealousy, and the unconsciousness
of others. Turtle teaches you, through its habit patterns, how to
use protection. If you are bothered by the actions or words of
others, it is time to go inside yourself and honor your feelings.
If you are attacked, it is time to give a warning snap.

If you have chosen the Turtle symbol, you are being asked
to honor the creative source within you, to be grounded to the
Earth, and to observe your situation with motherly compassion.
Use the water and earth energies, which represent Turtle's two
homes, to flow harmoniously with your situation and to place
your feet firmly on the ground in a power stance.

Turtle is a fine teacher of the art of grounding. You may
even be able to overcome some of your "space cadet" tendencies
if you align with Turtle medicine. In learning to ground, you are
placing focus on your thoughts and actions and slowing to a
pace that assures completion.

Turtle warns of the dangers of "pushing the river," as evidenced by the plodding pace it keeps. The corn that is harvested before its time is not yet full. However if it is given the chance to develop at its own rate, in its own season, its sweetness will be shared by all.

Turtle buries its thoughts, like its eggs, in the sand, and allows the Sun to hatch the little ones. This teaches you to develop your ideas before bringing them out in the light. Look at the old fable of the tortoise and the hare, and decide for yourself whether or not you would like to align with Turtle. Bigger, stronger, and faster are not always the best ways to get to a goal. When you arrive, you may be asked where you've been and you may not be able to remember. In that case, arriving prematurely can make you feel very immature.

If you draw the Turtle card, it augurs a time of connecting with the power of Earth and the Mother-Goddess within. This is a reminder of the ally you have in Mother Earth. It does not matter what situation you have created: ask her for assistance, and abundance will follow.

CONTRARY:

Pulling the Turtle card in the reverse means that Mother Earth is calling you to reconnect in some way. If you have become flippant and forgotten to place waste in its proper place instead of throwing it out the car window, she is calling. If you have felt alone in your time of need, she is calling. If you have been struggling financially or have little to eat, or if you have desired a child and see no pregnancy in the near future, she is your medicine — use it. You are not alone . . . ever. You are a child of Earth. All acts of pleasure, joy, and abundance are given by the Mother of the creative force. Use her energy to aid you, and you will be healed enough to share this energy with others.

The idea of a Turtle helplessly trying to right itself after it has been flipped upside down can also symbolize contrary Turtle. You are not a victim, and you are not helpless, no matter how much it may seem like this is the case in your present situation. To right the ill-dignified Turtle, you need only list the

things you are grateful for, and from that grateful place in your
heart, look for the abundance of alternatives that Mother
Earth gives.

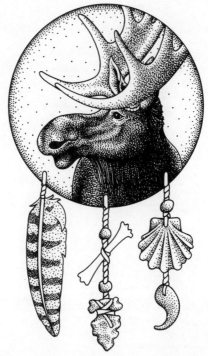

Moose . . .

Help me to honor the gifts I can give,
And recognize my worthiness long as I live.

11
Moose

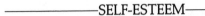

Moose is found in the North of the medicine wheel, as is Buffalo. North represents the place of wisdom. Self-esteem is the medicine of Moose because it represents the power of recognizing that wisdom has been used in a situation and that recognition or a pat on the back is deserved.

Moose is the largest member of the deer family, and has great strength. The call of the male Moose is an awesome thing to hear on a musky spring night. His pride in his maleness and his desire to share his seed with a Moose cow are displays of his sense of self-esteem. The bellow of a male Moose can be viewed as a positive force, since it represents his willingness to "tell the world" about his feelings.

This "tell the world" trait contains a joyfulness which only comes with a sense of accomplishment. There is no greater joy than a job well done. This trait is therefore not a seeking of approval, but rather an enjoyment of sharing because of the spontaneous explosion of joy that comes from the deepest part of one's being.

The wisdom woven throughout this scenario is that creation constantly brings forth new ideas and further creation. Moose is telling us that joy should be shouted with pride. The wisdom in doing this shouting is that the joy is "catching." In a sense, the bellowing is a way for all of us to lighten up and give ourselves or each other a "well done!"

Moose medicine people have the ability to know when to use the gentleness of Deer and when to activate the stampede of Buffalo. They understand the balance between giving orders to get things done and having a willingness to do things themselves. The wisdom of Moose medicine is akin to the Grandfather Warrior who has long since put away his war paint and is now advising the young bucks to cool their blood.

Moose medicine is often found in elders who have walked the Good Red Road and have seen many things in their Earth Walk. Their joy lies in being the teachers of the children, and in being the first ones to give encouragement. This is not to say that Moose medicine people do not use their wisdom to warn as well as to give praise, because they do. Moose medicine people know what to say, when to say it, and to whom.

The elders are honored in tribal law for their gifts of wisdom, for their teaching abilities, and for the calmness they impart in Council. If you are wise beyond your years and have the gift of Moose medicine, use this gift to encourage others to learn and grow. There are many facets to the wisdom of Moose medicine.

If you have chosen the Moose card, you have reason to feel good about something you have accomplished on your journey. This may be a habit you have broken, a completion of some sort, an insight on a goal, or a new sense of self that you have fought hard to earn. It is a time of feeling harmonious pride, and of recognizing those who aided you in the process.

One good exercise in Moose medicine is to write down things that you can love about yourself and your progress in life. Then apply these same things to friends, family, coworkers, and life. Don't forget to share the findings with others. They need the encouragement as much as you do.

CONTRARY:

If Moose is upside-down when you draw it, you are being reminded that ego can ruin your sense of accomplishment. Remember that others have the same potential you have, and do not become careless in your appreciation of their gifts. Reversed Moose implies that in tooting your own horn you have failed to be interested in others, and have therefore forgotten that everyone teaches everyone else in some way. Contrary Moose medicine may be asking you to grow quietly for awhile, to calm your spirit and allow the strength and wisdom of silence to enter your heart. This is the core of Moose medicine: knowing the wisdom of silence, so that when it is proper to speak you can take pride in your words.

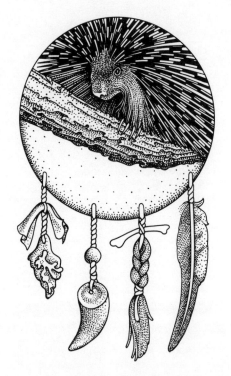

Porcupine . . . remind me,
Of innocence again,

With every man a brother,
Each woman a friend.

12
Porcupine

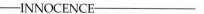

The South of the medicine wheel is the place of childlike innocence and humility. It is the home of playfulness, and the position of Porcupine on the medicine wheel of life.

Porcupine has many special qualities, and a very powerful medicine: the power of faith and trust. The power of faith contains within it the ability to move mountains. The power of trust in life involves trusting that the Great Spirit has a divine plan. Your task is to find the pathway that is most beneficial for you and that uses your greatest talents to further the plan. Trust can open doorways to the creation of space. The space thus created allows others to open their hearts to you and to share their gifts of love, joy, and companionship.

If you were to observe Porcupine, you would immediately notice its quills. These quills are only used when trust has been broken between Porcupine and another creature. Much like otter, Porcupine is a gentle, loving creature, and nonaggressive. When fear is not present, it is possible to feed a Porcupine by hand and never get stuck by its quills.

Through understanding the basic nature of this animal, you may come to understand your own need for trust and faith, and for becoming like a child again. In today's society, this is a needed reminder to honor the wonder of life and the appreciation of each new day as an adventure of discovery.

Porcupine sat silently, looking at a hollow log. She wondered if it was a playhouse that nature had created just for her. Porcupine envisioned all the things she could do with the log. She could climb on top and make the log roll from side to side. She could go inside and see if there were any juicy worms for her dinner. She could also scratch her back on the rough outer bark if she wanted to.

Just as Porcupine was pondering what to do next, she saw Bear approaching. Bear was big and black and looking for honey. "Oh, another playmate to share my log," she thought.

"Hello, Bear," she cooed. "Do you want to play and share my log with me?"

Gruff old Bear snorted, "Porcupine, don't you know that I'm too old to play? You're in my way. I'm looking for honey. Go away!"

"Why Bear, you're never too old to play," she replied. "If you forget what it was like to be a cub, you'll always be as impatient and gruff as you are now."

Bear began to think about what Porcupine had said. Maybe she was right. All the other creatures had run away from Bear in fright. Even the other Bears had turned up their noses when he growled at them. This little Porcupine was certainly trusting him not to eat her. She even offered to be his friend.

The old Bear looked at Porcupine and began to feel something move inside him. He started to remember the games he had played as a cub. Joy started to live in him again.

"Little Porcupine, you have reminded me that in becoming strong and seeking answers, I got caught in trying to be an intellectual. I became afraid of what others would think if I dropped my mask of gruffness. I was afraid they wouldn't take me seriously anymore. You have taught me that in being a fuddy-duddy, I was causing others not to care for me. Thank you. I'd love to play with this old log."

And so it was that Bear became childlike again and learned the innocence of Porcupine.

In choosing the Porcupine card, you have given yourself a gentle reminder not to get caught in the chaos of the adult world where fear, greed, and suffering are commonplace. The medicine in this card is that of relief from seriousness and severity. Open your heart to those things that gave you joy as a child. Remember the preciousness of fantasy and imagination, and the making of some game or toy from nothing but scraps.

Honor the playfulness of spirit that lets everyone win.

CONTRARY:

In pulling the Porcupine card reversed, you are giving your-self a timely warning that you cannot win the game of life if you are too serious. In some area of your life, you may be feeling hurt or afraid of trusting again. It is possible that life has recently dealt you a hard blow. If this is so, it is time to begin again by placing faith in your ability to overcome the lesson with joy. Are you willing to trust yourself? If so, you might begin by writing down the feelings that come out of the situation. How can you, as your adult-self, comfort you, the child within, and teach your inner child how to have faith and trust again?

The ill-dignified Porcupine is belly-up, with its quills stuck in the ground. This is a rather defenseless position. You may be forcing yourself to be vulnerable so that you can regain your hope. Perhaps you needed to roll over to get your tummy patted. This position could therefore indicate that you are ready to accept a little love from others. In any case, if you are not willing to trust again, this card is forcing you to look at why. Or at why not!

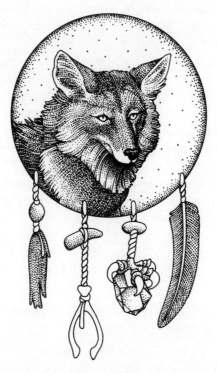

Coyote . . . you devil!
You tricked me once more!
Must I sit and ponder,
What you did it for?

13
Coyote

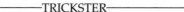

—————————TRICKSTER—————————

There are thousands of myths and stories about Coyote, the great trickster. Many Native cultures call Coyote the "Medicine Dog." If you have pulled this card, you can be sure that some kind of medicine is on its way — and it may or may not be to your liking. Whatever the medicine is, good or bad, you can be sure it will make you laugh, maybe even painfully. You can be sure that Coyote will teach you a lesson about yourself.

Coyote has many magical powers, but they do not always work in his favor. His own trickery fools him. He is the master trickster who tricks himself. No one is more astonished than Coyote at the outcome of his own tricks. He falls into his own trap. And yet he somehow manages to survive. He may be banged and bruised by the experience, but he soon goes on his way to even *greater error*, forgetting to learn from his mistakes. He may have lost the battle, but he is never beaten.

Coyote is sacred. In the folly of his acts we see our own foolishness. As Coyote moves from one disaster to the next, he refines the art of self-sabotage to sheer perfection. No one can blindly do themselves or others in with more grace and ease than this holy trickster. Coyote takes himself so seriously at times that he cannot see the obvious; for example, the steamroller that is about to run over him. That is why, when it hits him, he still cannot believe it. "Was that really a steamroller? I better go look," he says. And he is run over once more.

Contained within trickster medicine is the humor of the ages. The cosmic joke is not just on ourselves but on everyone else, if they are following Coyote or have strong Coyote medicine. Someone like this may be able to convince others that a skunk smells like roses, but the fact remains that it is still a skunk.

Snooze time is over if you have pulled the Coyote medicine card.
Watch out! Your glass house may crash to the ground at any moment. All your self-mirrors may shatter. The divine trickster is dog-
ging you, and you may trip. Coyote scratches under his arm. He
does a crazy dance. He catches his tail on fire playing with
matches. He jumps in the fishpond to save himself and nearly
drowns. Coyote seduces a concrete statue. Coyote thinks he has
found a bone, but it is a rattlesnake. Everyone watches the comedic
scene. Coyote is you, me, booby traps, jet airplanes with toilets that
don't work, blind dates, and all the humorous and whimsical things
we encounter along life's way. Get ready for more of the laughs —
lots more.

Go immediately beneath the surface of your experiences.
Ask yourself what you are really doing and why. Is Coyote your
medicine? Are you playing jokes on yourself? Are you trying to
fool an adversary? Is someone tricking you? Do you want to give
the office "geek" the phone number of the beautiful new
secretary? Or do you want to pull a prank on your best friend?
When was the last time you did something just because it was
crazy and fun?

On the other hand, you may not be conscious of your own
pathway of foolishness. You may have conned yourself, your family, your friends, or even the public at large into believing that you
know what you are doing. But listen, Coyote. You are balled up
in your own machinations. You have created a befuddling, be-
wildering, confounding *trick*. Pick up the juggler eyes from the
ground and put them back in their sockets. See through the genius
of your acts of self-sabotage. Find it amusing and laugh, trickster,
laugh.

If you can't laugh at yourself and your crazy antics, you have
lost the game. Coyote always comes calling when things get too serious. The medicine is in laughter and joking so that new viewpoints may be assumed.

If you have Coyote medicine, you may use it to make stuffy
old fogies lighten up, to add cheer to a party, or to break a "death-
grip conversation" with ease. Look at the positive side of sabotaging nosey questions about your personal life. Have *fun* telling

some gossiper that you just returned from St. Tropez in your new Lear Jet!

CONTRARY:

If Coyote appears in the reversed position, you can be assured that he is going to be contrary and a pain in your side. Look around yourself and watch which direction he is coming from. If Coyote is approaching you from the outside, beware of this master of illusion. Coyote may put you in his spell and take you to a briar patch to pick berries. It will be a painful lesson for you if you follow him. Coyote reversed can appear in your life as a supposed all-knowing teacher, a scam artist, a get-rich-quick business planner, a rare coin door-to-door salesperson, a femme fatale, a movie producer, a television evangelist, a swamp-land realtor, a politician, or anybody who wants you to follow their lead. Coyote is not the recommended business partner or lover.

Contrary Coyote may signal a time when everything you touch backfires. All your jokes may be exploding in your face. In this reversed position, Coyote also signals a time to be aware of the intentions of others, and to look for the boomerang *you* threw at another person coming back to knock you from behind. Someone else's trick may be on you, or there could be deception in the wind. Whatever Coyote reversed has conjured up, it could be coming from any direction. Remember, this joker is always wild!

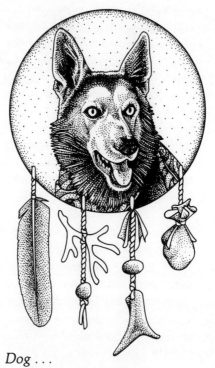

Dog . . .
    You are so noble,
    Until the bitter end,
    Your medicine is the teaching,
    Of true and loyal friends.

14
Dog

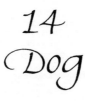

---LOYALTY---

All of the Southwest and Plains Indian tribes had Dogs. These noble animals would often give warning signals of approaching danger. They helped in the hunt and were a great source of warmth on long winter nights. Since the canine tribe has many breeds, early Indian Dogs were usually half-wild. This wildness, however, never divested the owners of their Dogs' innate loyalty.

Dog has been considered the servant of humanity throughout history. If a person carries Dog medicine, he or she is usually serving others or humanity in some way. Here you will find the charity worker, the philanthropist, the nurse, the counselor, the minister, and the soldier.

Dog was the servant-soldier that guarded the tribe's lodges from surprise attack. Dog is a medicine that embodies the loving gentleness of *best friend* and the half-wild *protector energy* of territorial imperative. Like Anubis, the jackal dog protector of Egypt, Dog is a guardian. Throughout history, Dog has been the guardian of hell, as well as of ancient secrets, hidden treasures, and babies—while mothers were cooking or in the fields. Dog honors its gifts and is loyal to the trust placed in its care.

In examining Dog medicine, you might find that you have fond personal memories of owning and loving Dog as a pet. The message that Dog is trying to give you is that you must delve deeply into your sense of service to others. Canines are genuinely service-oriented animals, and are devoted to their owners with a sense of loyalty that supersedes how they are treated.

If Dog has been yelled at or paddled, it still returns love to the person who was the source of its bad treatment. This does not come from stupidity, but rather from a deep and compassionate understanding of human shortcomings. It is as if a tolerant spirit dwells in the heart of every canine that asks only to be of service.

You can also see Dogs that have had the loyalty beaten out of them. They cower and cry at the slightest look of disapproval, but this is not their normal nature. Some varieties of Dogs have even been trained against their natures to be brutal and vicious. Out of a sense of service, these breeds have adopted the attack-oriented desires of their owners. They carry an altered genetic memory of what service means if they are to be approved of by their masters.

Dog medicine asks you to look at how readily your sense of loyalty is countermanded by your need for approval. If you have pulled the Dog card, there are several questions you need to consider, depending on the situation about which you are asking.

1) Have I recently forgotten that I owe my allegiance to my personal truth in life?

2) Is it possible that gossip or the opinions of others have jaded my loyalty to a certain friend or group?

3) Have I denied or ignored someone who is trying to be my loyal friend?

4) Have I been loyal and true to my goals?

CONTRARY:

In the contrary position, Dog may be telling you that you have become critical or mean due to the company you are keeping. The reversal of this medicine could also imply that it is time to stop cowering with fear, and time to begin to tackle the adversaries of your confidence. The key is to realize that these are not external enemies, but thought-forms in your own mind which tell you that you are not worthy of loyalty — either to yourself or to others. You may want to examine the patterns of disloyalty in your life. Do you, for example, pass on gossip, or not speak up when someone else is rumor-mongering? Do you make jokes that belittle others? Do you refuse to return kindness? These are characteristics of fear, and particularly of a fear that is common to the human, two-legged family: the fear of not belonging or of not being approved of.

Reclaim the power of loyalty to self and self truths. Become like Dog — your own best friend.

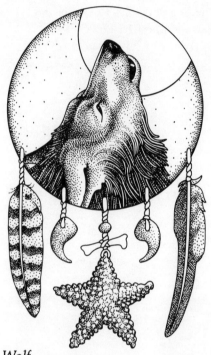

Wolf . . .
   Teacher,
      Pathfinder,
         Moon-dog of my soul.

Howling,
   Singing,
      Teaching how to know.

15
Wolf

---TEACHER---

Wolf is the pathfinder, the forerunner of new ideas who returns to the clan to teach and share medicine. Wolf takes one mate for life and is loyal like Dog. If you were to keep company with Wolves, you would find an enormous sense of family within the pack, as well as a strong individualistic urge. These qualities make Wolf very much like the human race. As humans we also have an ability to be a part of society and yet still embody our individual dreams and ideas.

In the Great Star Nation, Wolf is represented by the Dog Star, Sirius, which legend tells us was the original home of our teachers in ancient times. Sirius was thought to be the home of the gods by the ancient Egyptians, and is still considered so by the Dogan tribe in Africa. It stands to reason that Native American peoples would formulate this same connection and adopt Wolf people as the clan of teachers.

The senses of Wolf are very keen, and the Moon is its power ally. The Moon is the symbol for psychic energy, or the unconscious that holds the secrets of knowledge and wisdom. Baying at the Moon may be an indication of Wolf's desire to connect with new ideas which are just below the surface of consciousness. Wolf medicine empowers the teacher within us all to come forth and aid the children of Earth in understanding the Great Mystery and life.

If you have drawn Wolf's card, you may be able to share your personal medicine with others. Your intuitive side may also have an answer or teaching for your personal use at this time. As you feel Wolf coming alive within you, you may wish to share your knowledge by writing or lecturing on information that will help others better understand their uniqueness or path in life. It is in the sharing of great truths that the consciousness of humanity will attain new heights. Wolf could also be telling you to seek out lonely places that will allow you to see your teacher within. In the aloneness of a power place, devoid of other humans, you may find the true you. Look for teachings no matter where you are. Wolf would not come to you unless you requested the appearance of the tribe's greatest teacher.

CONTRARY:

If Wolf is reversed, you are being asked to expand your limited view of the present situation. Doing this may entail a great deal of courage and a willingness to look at new ideas. It could also require that you delete some old ideas to make room for the expansiveness that always comes when you are willing to learn. The gift of wisdom comes to you when you have walked enough pathways and found enough dead ends to truly know the forest. In the discovery and rediscovery of every inch of ground comes the knowledge that nothing ever remains the same.

Contrary Wolf may also be telling you that stagnation or fear of asserting your viewpoint has bogged down the flow of change in your life. Wolf reversed is *always* urging you to seek the teachers or pathfinders that will show you the way to new life experiences. Remember, the teacher or pathfinder may be the small still voice within, as well as a person, a leaf, a cloud, a stone, a tree, a book, or the Great Spirit.

To live is to grow, and growing comes through accepting all life forms as your teachers. Become Wolf, and take up the sense of adventure. You may just stop howling and learn to *become* the moon.

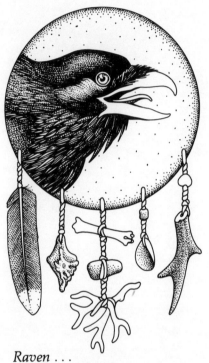

Raven . . .
   Black as pitch,
      Mystical as the moon,

Speak to me of magic,
   I will fly with you soon.

16
Raven

Throughout time, Raven has carried the medicine of magic. This has been true in many cultures across the planet. It is sacred, in the medicine ways, to honor Raven as the bringer of magic. If the magic is bad medicine, the carrier may be honored out of fear rather than out of respect. Those who fear Raven may do so because they have been dabbling in areas in which they had no knowledge, and a spell may have backfired on them. Rather than analyzing the dark side of sorcery, realize that you will fear Raven only if you need to learn about your inner fears or self-created demons.

Raven magic is a powerful medicine that can give you the courage to enter the darkness of the void, which is the home of all that is not yet in form. The void is called the Great Mystery. Great Mystery existed before all other things came into being. Great Spirit lives inside the void and emerged from the Great Mystery. Raven is the messenger of the void.

If Raven appears in your spread, you are about to experience a change in consciousness. This may involve walking inside the Great Mystery on another path at the edge of time. It would portend a signal brought by the Raven that says, "You have earned the right to see and experience a little more of life's magic." Raven's color is the color of the void — the black hole in space that holds all the energy of the creative source.

In Native teachings the color black means many things, but it does not mean evil. Black can mean the seeking of answers, the void, or the road of the spiritual or nonphysical. The blue-black of Raven contains an iridescence that speaks of the magic of darkness, and a changeability of form and shape that brings an awakening in the process.

Raven is the guardian of ceremonial magic and *in absentia* healing. In any healing circle, Raven is present. Raven guides the magic of healing and the change in consciousness that will bring about a new reality and dispel "dis-ease" or illness. Raven brings in the new state of wellness from the Void of Great Mystery and the field of plenty.

Raven is the messenger that carries all energy flows of ceremonial magic between the ceremony itself and the intended destination. For instance, if a ceremony is being performed to send energy to a disaster area where people need courage and strength, Raven would be the courier for that energy flow. The intention could be to allow the people of the devastated area to feel the concern and support of the participants in the ceremony.

If you have chosen Raven, magic is in the air. Do not try to figure it out; you cannot. It is the power of the unknown at work, and something special is about to happen. The deeper mystery, however, is how you will respond to the sparkling synchronicity of this alchemical moment. Will you recognize it and use it to further enhance your growth? Can you accept it as a gift from the Great Spirit? Or will you limit the power of the Great Mystery by explaining it away?

It may be time to call Raven as a courier to carry an intention, some healing energy, a thought, or a message. Raven is the patron of smoke signals or spirit messages represented by smoke. So if you want to send a message to the Blue Road of spirit, in order to contact the Ancients, call Raven. Or, who knows, the Ancients may be calling to you.

Remember, this magic moment came from the void of darkness, and the challenge is to bring it to light. In doing so you will have honored the magician within.

CONTRARY:

Raven reversed is not to be taken lightly! It can mean that the boomerang is coming home. If you have wished harm to another, beware — you have asked for this harm to teach you in turn what it feels like. If you have not been wishing evil on another, contrary Raven may be bringing you a warning that you are not equipped to move into another level of consciousness until you have mastered the one you are currently working with. On yet another level, Raven may be telling you that you have forgotten the magic of life and have settled into a mundane rut. If this rut suits you and you do not want to experience the extraordinary magic in your life, ask Raven to fly through your dreams and give you a taste of its medicine. If you do, you may never be the same again.

Contrary Raven may also portend a time of smoky, confused messages that you cannot see or hear because your "intellect" is insisting that magic is not real. If you cannot imagine or pretend due to your lack of faith in magic or miracles, healing cannot take place. Raven may be pecking at the door to your consciousness, but you will not receive unless you clear the smoke and seek the other realms of imagination and awareness where magic lives.

To right the contrary Raven, you may need to seek a trained shaman to clear the energy field you have created. You might need to block some negative energy sent by another person, or cancel the harm you wished on someone else. Keep it clean! This is the message when the magic moves into smoky shadow. Seek healing and a clearing of intention, then reach for the stars and honor Mother Earth and all other living things. Fill yourself with the magic of being alive and call Raven to teach you the proper way of using energy. Ground that energy so that manifestation of the magic can occur. Do this in love and simplicity. Raven will tell you this magical truth: Never go beyond that which you have prepared and trained for. Life is good, so use the magic to aid the entire family of Earth.

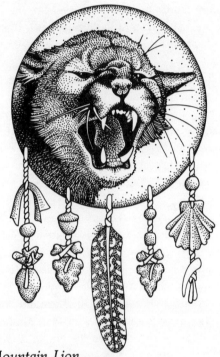

Mountain Lion . . .
  Oh kingly leader,
    Of sleek, feline form,

Touch my heart with courage,
  Then sound the alarm,

That I may lead with foresight,
  Assurance bright and true,
    To carry on the spirit,
      Of the strength I see in you.

17
Mountain Lion

—————————LEADERSHIP—————————
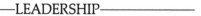

Mountain Lion can be a very difficult power totem for you
to have, because it places you in a position to be a target for
the problems of others. You could be blamed for things going
wrong, or for always taking charge when others cannot. You
could become the perfect justification for the insecurities
of others.

Mountain Lion medicine involves lessons on the use of
power in leadership. It is the ability to lead without insisting
that others follow. It is the understanding that all beings are
potential leaders in their own ways. The use and abuse of power
in a position of influence are part of this great cat's medicine.

By observing the graceful pounce of Mountain Lion, you
will learn how to balance power, intention, physical strength,
and grace. This relates, in human terms, to the balance of body,
mind, and spirit. The giant feline never wastes anything. It only
kills what it needs for survival. The female lion is the hunter
who graces her table in a style akin to mother energy.

If Mountain Lion has come to you in dreams, it is a time to
stand on your convictions and lead yourself where your heart
takes you. Others may choose to follow, and the lessons will
multiply. If you have pulled the card of Mountain Lion, you
may be asked to review the purpose behind your personal beliefs.
You may need to discover whether or not your plans include a
pride of cubs wanting to be like you or to share in your dreams.
If you are already a leader, the question may be whether or not
the time has come to push the cubs out of the cave. If you are
aligned with cat medicine, you are considered to be "king of the
mountain," and never allowed to be human or vulnerable. The
pitfalls are many, but the rewards are great.

In assuming the place of power that Mountain Lion affords, you must constantly be aware of keeping peace. However you can never make everyone happy unless you lie to yourself or others. This is human nature. Therefore the first responsibility of leadership is to tell the truth. Know it and live it, and your example will filter down to the tiniest cub in the pride. *Responsibility* is no more than the *ability to respond* to any situation. Panic is not a part of this sacred medicine.

CONTRARY:

If your Mountain Lion card is reversed, you may be playing with fire. A leader who tries to lead through tyranny or dictatorship has forgotten the medicine of truth. Through the reversal of this medicine, you may be tricked into believing that nothing else has validity except the ideas created by yourself. Watch out! Rome crumbled for this very reason! If this aspect of the contrary medicine does not apply to your situation, look at other messages which Mountain Lion brings in the reversed position.

If you are avoiding taking your place of leadership, it could be because the whole idea scares you silly. This is a normal state of affairs for one who has never been a leader before. In this instance it is necessary to call upon the courage of Lion and to begin by learning the lessons of the "lion-hearted."

Another message of Mountain Lion reversed is to not let yourself be led down the primrose path by a leader who is abusing power. If you want to put yourself on the road to being a leader in your own right, ask questions of anyone to whom you have given authority. See if they carry the medicine of Mountain Lion, and whether you can grow into your own leadership by observing how they handle the task of setting examples.

Become Mountain Lion by refusing to hide in the cave of your own shyness or uncertainty. Roar with conviction, roar with power, and remember to roar with laughter to balance the medicine!

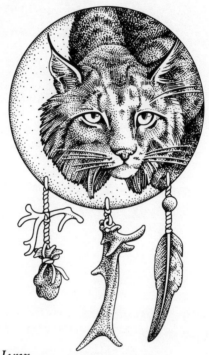

Lynx . . .
> *You know the secrets*
>> *So very well,*
> *The Dreamtime and the magic,*
>> *But you'll never tell.*

May I learn to hold my tongue,
> *Observe like the Sphinx,*
>> *Powerful, yet silent,*
>>> *The medicine of Lynx.*

18
Lynx

It is said that if you want to find out a secret, ask Lynx medicine. Unfortunately, it is difficult to get the silent Lynx to speak. To be confronted by the powerful medicine of Lynx signifies that you do not know something about yourself or others.

Lynx is the keeper of the secrets of lost magical systems and occult knowledge. Lynx has the ability to move through time and space, and to go into the Great Silence for unravelling any mystery. Lynx is not the *guardian* of secrets, but the *knower* of secrets. The problem lies in getting Lynx to instruct you. He or she would rather be off chasing a bird or kicking sand in your face than running circles around you.

Lynx medicine is a very specific type of clairvoyance. If this medicine is strong in you, you will get mental pictures concerning other people and the exact things they have hidden, either from themselves or from others. You will see their fears, their lies, and their self-deceptions. You will also know where they have hidden the treasure, if there is any. You never speak of these revelations—you simply know.

The only way you can coax information about yourself out of a Lynx medicine person (in case you have forgotten where you hid the treasure) is to respect the practices of his or her tradition. If you go to a Gypsy with Lynx medicine, you must show your respect by *paying* with money after the reading. If you go to a Choctaw medicine person, he or she will reach into your midsection, or use other traditional methods to help you. A blanket or tobacco should be given in exchange for the medicine he or she has performed for you. This maxim is known as the law of the Lynx people, and is practiced by Native American, Gypsy, Sufi, and Egyptian cultures, among others.

If you have pulled the Lynx card, you can be sure that "secrets" are afloat. If this is your personal medicine, you should listen to your higher self. Be still and pay attention to the revelations you receive either in the form of mental pictures or through a high singing voice in your inner ear. Perhaps you will receive information in the form of omens. You can be sure that Mother Earth is signalling to you in some manner.

If Lynx is at your door, listen. Brother or Sister Lynx can teach you of your personal power and of things you have forgotten about yourself. Lynx can lead you to lost treasures, and connect you to forgotten brotherhoods or sisterhoods.

Some medicine people believe that the Sphinx of ancient Egypt was not a Lion but a Lynx. This Lynx does not say much. With an enigmatic smile, the great cat watches over the sands of forever.

CONTRARY:

If Lynx has appeared in the reversed position, it is time to shut your big mouth. Something you are jabbering about has let the "cat" out of the bag. Are you defiling a sacred trust, or have you broken a promise to a friend? If not, you may have pulled a good prank on yourself by blabbing your latest idea to the friend of a competitor. Watch your tongue and see if you are able to refrain from gossiping, or talking about your latest romantic conquest. Look and see if, in your present state, you are able to listen and truly be interested in someone else's stories or ideas. On this level, Lynx is telling you to become worthy of trust. Then the secrets will be available to you.

You might look at choosing to have your brain in gear before your babble starts, or your foot may have to replace your tongue. This is the "know it all" syndrome. Fine — if you want to talk, just sew up your ears. After all, talking leaves no room for hearing or learning. Lynx is a tough teacher, and if you have let the cat out of the bag, be ready for the consequences.

Become Lynx and wear the Mona Lisa smile. Only you will

know what you are smiling about. The cat will not have your tongue — you will — as well as the power over it.

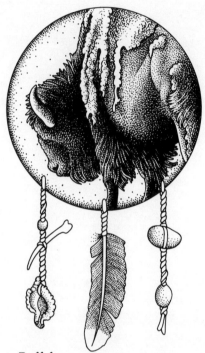

Buffalo . . .
    You bring us,
        The gifts of life.

Hear our prayers,
    Smoke rising,
        Like Phoenix,

We are reborn,
    Within the sacred words.

19
Buffalo

————PRAYER & ABUNDANCE————

In the Lakota tradition it was the White Buffalo Calf Woman who brought the sacred pipe to the people and taught them to pray. The bowl of the pipe was the receptacle that held tobacco, an herb with male and female medicine. The stem of the pipe represented the male entering the female and seeding life. In the coming together of male and female, the connection to the divine energy of the Great Spirit was made. As the pipe was loaded with tobacco, every family in nature was asked to enter into the pipe and share its medicine as prayer and praise to the heavens. The smoke was considered to be visual prayer, and was very sacred and cleansing.

All animals are sacred, but in many traditions White Buffalo is the most sacred. The appearance of White Buffalo is a sign that prayers are being heard, that the sacred pipe is being honored, and that the promises of prophesy are being fulfilled. White Buffalo signals a time of abundance and plenty.

Buffalo was the major source of sustenance for the Plains Indians. It gave meat for food, hides for clothing, warm and soft buffalo robes for long winters, and hooves for glue. The medicine of Buffalo is prayer, gratitude and praise for that which has been received. Buffalo medicine is also knowing that *abundance* is present when all relations are honored as sacred, and when gratitude is expressed to every living part of creation.

Because of its desire to give the gifts that its body provided, and because of its willingness to be used on Earth for the highest good before entering the hunting grounds of Spirit, Buffalo did not readily stampede and run from hunters.

To use Buffalo medicine is to smoke the pipe in a sacred manner, and to give praise for the richness of life to be shared with all races, all creatures, all nations, and all life. It means smoking for others so that their needs are met, praying for the good of all things in harmony, and accepting the Great Mystery as a part of that harmony.

If you have drawn the Buffalo card, you may be asked to use your energy in prayer. You may also be called upon to be an instrument of someone else's answer to a prayer. This could portend a time of recognizing the sacredness of every walk of life, albeit different from your own. To honor another's pathway, even if it brings you sadness, is a part of the message that Buffalo brings. This may be a time of reconnection to the meaning of life and the value of peace. Most assuredly this time will bring serenity amidst chaos if you pray in earnest for enlightenment and the power of calmness and give praise for the gifts you already have.

Buffalo medicine is a sign that you achieve nothing without the aid of the Great Spirit and that you must be humble enough to ask for that assistance and then be grateful for what you receive.

CONTRARY:

To receive Buffalo upside-down is a signal that you have forgotten to seek help when it has been needed. If your hand is closed in a fist, you cannot receive the bounty of abundance. In understanding the significance of the reversed Buffalo, you may well ask yourself.

1) Have I forgotten my eternal partner, the Great Spirit?

2) Am I pushing myself too fast in the physical world and keeping myself from seeing the importance of reunion with the Source of all life?

3) Have I forgotten to honor the ways of others and to afford them the same respect that I wish to receive for myself?

4) Am I feeling like my life is being used for the highest good at this time?

5) Have I forgotten to be grateful for my life, my possessions, my talents, my abilities, my health, my family, or my friends?

6) Is it time to make peace with another, or to make peace with some inner conflict I have so that I may walk in balance again?

Become Buffalo. Feel the smoke of prayer and praise change your Buffalo robe to white so that you may be an answer to the prayers of the world.

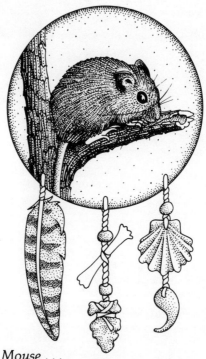

Mouse . . .

> If I could see the world,
> Through your tiny eyes,
> Maybe then I would know,
> How to scrutinize.
>
> Every detail carries weight,
> And true to its purpose,
> Has its perfect puzzle place,
> To stop the "three-ring circus!"

20
Mouse

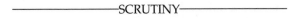

————————SCRUTINY————————

Mouse says, "I will touch everything with my whiskers in order to know it." Paradoxically, this is both a great power and a great weakness. It is good medicine to see up close. It is good medicine to pay attention to detail, but it is bad medicine to chew every little thing to pieces.

Mouse has many predatory enemies, including birds, snakes, and cats. Since Mouse is food for many, it has a highly developed sense of danger at every turn. So-called civilization is a highly complex set of components which calls for more and more organizational skills and scrutiny to detail every year. Mouse is a powerful medicine to have in these modern times. Things that might appear insignificant to others take on enormous importance to Mouse.

Mouse people anger many other medicine types because they appear to be nit-pickers. Mouse people will spot the lint on your coat, even if it matches in color. They will try to convince you that the simplest task is fraught with difficulty. They are fixated on methodology. They sort and categorize and file away for later use. They may seem like they are hoarding, but this is the farthest thing from Mouse's mind. They are merely putting everything in order so that they will be able to explore it more carefully at a later date.

The chiefs tell us that without Mouse there would be no systemization of knowledge. Mouse ended Renaissance man and harkened the age of specialization. Mouse knew from the very beginning that "there is always more to learn." One can always delve deeper and deeper and deeper.

If your personal medicine is Mouse, you may be fearful of life but very well organized, with a compartment for everything.

You should try to see a larger picture than the one staring you in the face. Develop largesse of spirit. Try to become aware of the Great Dance of Life. Realize that even though you may be sitting in Los Angeles, there is also a New York, a Moon, a solar system, a galaxy, and an infinite universe. Jump high, little friend. You will glimpse the Sacred Mountain.

If mouse is in your card-spread, its medicine is telling you to *scrutinize*. Look at yourself and others carefully. Maybe that big hunk of cheese is sitting on a trigger that will spring a deadly trap. Maybe the cat is in the pantry waiting for you. Maybe someone to whom you have delegated authority, such as a doctor, a lawyer, or even a plumber, is not doing the job faithfully. The message is to see what is right before your eyes and to take action accordingly.

CONTRARY:

Mouse in the contrary position may be telling you that you are spending too much time with matters of great consequence when you should be paying a traffic ticket or sweeping the hogan. You may have let yourself become slovenly. You may have developed a disdain for authority and order. You may be procrastinating about something that needs immediate attention. Bring Mouse medicine to your life's chaos and you will soon have everything tidy and shipshape.

Another message of Mouse reversed may be that you are "pipe dreaming" about your own importance in life. Are you wondering why you have not been nominated for an Academy Award? You can't be recognized if you are not taking care of life's details and walking in humility. Remember that all good things come to those willing to work toward wholeness. Little Mouse needs to see the big picture, but only assimilate the information the picture gives a little at a time. Expansiveness can be overwhelming if you forget to take it step by step. Confusion is a product of "too much, too soon." Little mouse can conquer any task by using its scrutiny. Slow down and right the contrary medicine. Stop chasing your tail or being confused by the maze and start observing the details of your present pathway.

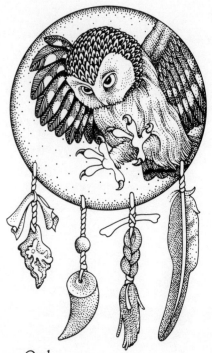

Owl . . .
   Magic,
      Omens,
         Time and space.

Does the truth emerge?
   Casting out deception,
      Silent flight,

Sacred Medicine Bird.

21
Owl

Owl medicine is symbolically associated with clairvoyance, astral projection, and magic, both black and white. Owl is called *Night Eagle* on several medicine wheels used by Amerindian teachers. Traditionally, Owl sits in the East, the place of illumination. Since time immemorial, humanity has been afraid of the night, the dark, and the unseen — waiting fearfully for the first crack of morning light. Conversely, night is Owl's friend.

Owl hunts its prey at night. Not only can Owl see in the dark, it can also accurately pinpoint and identify any sound. This gives it a great advantage when seeking food. Owls are the night hunters. Some Native people are fearful of Owl and call its feathers "deceiver feathers." An Owl feather is silent. You cannot hear Owl when it flies, but its prey definitely knows when it strikes, for its beak and talons are razor sharp.

Owl is oftentimes the medicine of sorcerers and witches. If Owl is your medicine, you will be drawn to magical practices and perhaps explore the dark arts. You should resist any temptation to practice black magic or *any* art that takes energy away from another person or being. If you have Owl medicine, these night birds will have a tendency to collect around you, even in the daytime, because they recognize a kinship with you.

Is it any wonder that in many cultures Owl is a symbol for wisdom? This is because Owl can see that which others cannot, which is the essence of true wisdom. Where others are deceived, Owl sees and knows what is there.

Athena, the Greek goddess of wisdom, had a companion Owl on her shoulder which revealed unseen truths to her. Owl had the ability to light up Athena's blind side, enabling her to speak the whole truth, as opposed to only a half truth.

If Owl is your personal medicine, no one can deceive you about what they are doing, no matter how they try to disguise or hide it from you. You may be a little frightening to be around, since so many people have ulterior motives which you see right through. If you are unaware of your medicine power, you may take your keen insights and abilities for granted. Others never do. You may frighten them and reflect their blindness, for you cannot be fooled. Owl medicine people know more about an individual's inner life than that person knows about herself or himself.

If you have pulled the Owl card, you are being asked to use your powers of keen, silent observation to intuit some life situation. Owl is befriending you and aiding you in seeing the total truth. Owl can bring you messages in the night through dreams or meditation. Pay attention to the signals and omens. The truth always brings further enlightenment.

CONTRARY:

If you have Owl upside-down in your cards, you have been greatly deceived by either yourself or another. Perhaps witch-craft or black magic is being used against you, or maybe you are using witchcraft or sorcery to aid you when you should be praying and asking the Great Spirit for guidance. The message is to befriend the darkness inside yourself. Look deeply, and soon the bright light of dawn will illuminate you. Then ask yourself what you are in the dark about. How and by whom are you being deceived? Have you lied to *yourself* about someone or something? Are you being greatly deceived, or just slightly deceived? Owl tells you to keep an eye on your property and your loved ones. Remember that Owl is always asking, "Who?"

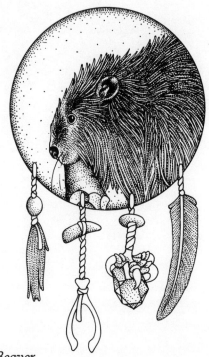

Beaver . . .
   Teach me to build my dreams,
      Including others too.

One mind,
   One thought,
      Hearts as one,
         Lessons learned from you.

22
Beaver

---BUILDER---

Beaver is the *doer* in the animal kingdom. Beaver medicine is akin to water and earth energy, and incorporates a strong sense of family and home. If you were to look at the dams that block woodland streams, you would find several entrances and exits. In building its home, Beaver always leaves itself many alternative escape routes. This practice is a lesson to all of us not to paint ourselves into corners. If we eliminate our alternatives, we dam the flow of experience in our lives. A doer is characterized by industriousness, and Beaver knows that limitation cancels productivity.

Beaver is armed with very sharp teeth that are capable of felling whole trees. Imagine what those teeth could do to the limbs of predators. From the rear, Beaver is armed with a paddle-like tail that aids in swimming as well as in guarding its behind. This tiny mammal is well equipped to protect its creation.

To understand Beaver medicine, you might take a look at the power of working and attaining a sense of achievement. In building a dream, teamwork is necessary. To accomplish a goal with others involves working with the group mind. Group mind constitutes harmony of the highest order, without individual egos getting in the way. Each partner in the project honors the talents and abilities of the others, and knows how to complete the piece of the puzzle that belongs to them. In working well with others, a sense of community is achieved and unity ensues.

If Beaver has appeared in your spread, it may be time to put your ideas into action or to complete some project that has been neglected. The Beaver card could also be asking you to settle differences with fellow workers or friends. Beaver tells you to look for alternative solutions to life's challenges and to protect the creations which you put your love and energy into.

Sometimes Beaver brings you a warning to watch your back. If this is your message, you will know it by the position in which the card falls in your spread. If the card falls in the South position, it is to remind your child-self that trusting is okay but caution is necessary. Use discernment and all will be fine.

CONTRARY:

If Beaver has dunked its head under water and is contrary, you are being asked to open new doors to opportunity and to stay aware. This could also usher in a time of laziness or apathy. Find what is damming the flow, and remove the impasse. The questions that may arise when Beaver is contrary are:

1) Have I forgotten to allow room in my life for new experiences?

2) Am I willing to work with others?

3) Am I resentful of having to work?

4) Do I express my creativity by doing, or just by dreaming about it?

5) Has my mind created so many obstacles to productivity that I feel like a failure before I begin?

Meditate upon Beaver's determination and willingness to work. Visualize the goal you wish to accomplish, and be willing to work with others to achieve that end.

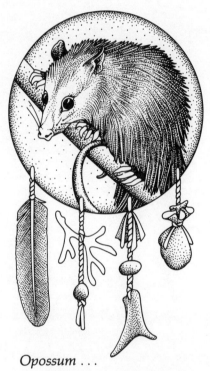

Opossum . . .
    Roll over!
        Are you really dead?

Or just playing Possum?

    Was it something I said?

23
Opossum

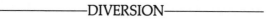

Opossum's greatest form of protection is to play dead. In doing this Opossum confuses many a predator into believing that the game is over. Oftentimes the confused rival walks away or looks the other direction for a moment, and Opossum runs to safety.

Opossum medicine uses a great deal of strategy. If all else fails, Opossum plays dead. It has the ability to fight with its claws and teeth, but it rarely uses this form of protection. Instead, the supreme strategy of diversion is constantly employed when things get a little too hard to handle. Opossum has developed an act that would receive an Academy Award in the animal kingdom. The musk of the death scent is excreted at will, adding to the master play that sends enemies on many trails of confusion.

If Opossum has turned up in your cards, you are being asked to use strategy in some present situation. Rely upon your instincts for the best way out of a tight corner. If you have to pretend to be apathetic or unafraid, do it! Oftentimes if you refuse to struggle or show that hurtful words bother you, your taunter will see no further fun in the game. Warriors have used Opossum medicine for centuries, playing dead when the enemy nears and outnumbers them. Then, in a flash, when the enemy is least expecting it, the war cry is heard. The fright of this serves to further confuse the unsuspecting opposition. Victory is sweet when the strategy is one of mental as well as physical prowess.

Opossum may be relaying to you that you are to expect the unexpected and be clever in achieving your victory. This could be a victory over a bothersome salesman or a nosey neighbor. In essence, Opossum is beckoning you to use your brain, your sense of drama, and surprise — to leap over some barrier to your progress.

CONTRARY:

In the reversed position, Opossum may be warning you against getting caught in the high drama of your life's present scenario. "Close your eyes and dramatize," may keep you from seeing the truth of a situation. You may buy into melodrama in yourself or others. You might as well play dead if you are justifying what you are doing with a tragic victim routine. If this concept does not apply to your situation, take a look at the possibility that you may have recently been giving excuses for why you don't want to do something instead of telling the truth. In fearing to hurt someone's feelings you may have trapped yourself in a justification pattern: "I'm too sick, I'm too poor, I'm watching my weight, I'm too short, tall, sad, busy, tired, etc."

In having to defend yourself with excuses, you may have lost the point. *You don't have to defend your right to be!* The exercise is in learning to politely say that something would not be appropriate for you at this time. That's all! You owe no one an excuse. Learn to imitate Opossum and play dead, in the sense that the best strategy is no defense. In assuming the viewpoint of no defense, you have chosen the right to be who and what you are with no games involved.

The proper use of diversion is to know when you do not need to use diversion at all. You owe no one an excuse for how you feel or what you choose to experience.

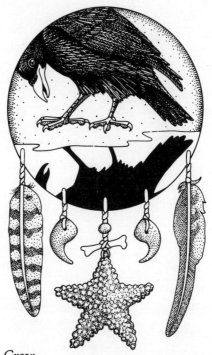

Crow . . .
    Are you "cawing,"
      So I may know,
        The secrets of balance,
          Within my soul?

    Or are you sending,
      Your sacred "caw"
        Just to remind me,
          Of universal laws?

24
Crow

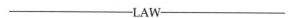

-------------------LAW-------------------

There is a medicine story that tells of Crow's fascination with her own shadow. She kept looking at it, scratching it, pecking at it, until her shadow woke up and became alive. Then Crow's shadow ate her. Crow is Dead Crow now.

Dead Crow is the Left-Handed Guardian. If you look deeply into Crow's eye, you will have found the gateway to the supernatural. Crow knows the unknowable mysteries of creation and is the keeper of all sacred law.

Since Crow is the keeper of sacred law, Crow can *bend* the laws of the physical universe and "shape shift." This ability is rare and unique. Few adepts exist in today's world, and fewer still have mastered Crow's art of shape shifting. This art includes doubling, or being in two places at one time *consciously*; taking on another physical form, and becoming the "fly on the wall" to observe what is happening far away.

The Europeans that came to Turtle Island were named the "boat people" by Slow Turtle. Even with the knowledge of alchemy possessed by certain boat people, none had ever seen the powerful shape shifting of shamans who utilized Crow medicine. Many boat people were frightened by what appeared to be animals coming into their camps or dwellings to discern their medicine. Crow medicine people are masters of illusion.

All sacred texts are under the protection of Crow. Creator's *Book of Laws* or *Book of Seals* is bound in Crow feathers. Crow feathers tell of spirit made flesh. Crow is also the protector of the "ogallah" or ancient records.

The Sacred Law Belts, or Wampum Belts, beaded by Native women long before the boat people or Europeans came to this continent, contain knowledge of the Great Spirit's laws, and are kept in the Black Lodges, the lodges of women. The law which states that "all things are born of women" is signified by Crow.

Children are taught to behave according to the rules of a particular culture. Most orthodox religious systems create a mandate concerning acceptable behavior within the context of worldly affairs. Do this and so, and you will go to heaven. Do thus and so, and you will go to hell. Different formulas for salvation are demanded by each "true faith."

Human law is not the same as Sacred Law. More so than any other medicine, Crow sees that the physical world and even the spiritual world, as humanity interprets them, are an illusion. There are billions of worlds. There are an infinitude of creatures. Great Spirit is within all. If an individual obeys Crow's perfect laws as given by the Creator, then at death he or she dies a Good Medicine death — going on to the next incarnation with a clear memory of his or her past.

Crow is an omen of change. Crow lives in the void and has no sense of time. The Ancient Chiefs tell us that Crow sees simultaneously the three fates — past, present and future. Crow merges light and darkness, seeing both inner and outer reality.

If Crow medicine appears in your card spread, you must pause and reflect on how you see the laws of the Great Spirit in relation to the laws of humanity. Crow medicine signifies a firsthand knowledge of a higher order of right and wrong than that indicated by the laws created in human culture. With Crow medicine, you speak in a powerful voice when addressing issues that for you seem out of harmony, out of balance, out of whack, or unjust.

Remember that Crow looks at the world with first one eye, and then the other—cross-eyed. In the Mayan culture, cross-eyeds had the privilege and duty of looking into the future. You must put aside your fear of being a voice in the wilderness and "caw" the shots as you see them.

As you learn to allow your *personal integrity* to be your guide, your sense of feeling alone will vanish. Your *personal will* can then emerge so that you will stand in your truth. The prime path of true Crow people says to be mindful of your opinions and actions. Be willing to walk your talk, speak your truth, know your life's mission, and balance past, present, and future in the now. Shape shift that old reality and become your future self. Allow the bending of physical laws to aid in creating the shape shifted world of peace.

CONTRARY:

So you are an outlaw today, eh? This is one of the varied messages of Crow reversed. The rebel in you has given a yell, and all hell is about to break loose!

A word to the wise at this point: Make sure that if you are stepping on toes, you have some back-up. The catalyst for a barroom brawl is usually the person with two black eyes. That is what it means to *eat* Crow.

If you do not plan to go to such extremes, Crow reversed may indicate that you are merely "cheating a little" on your diet, or covertly watching the neighbors have a spat, or thinking, "Promises are made to be broken." In any of these situations, the only loser is you. If you are lying to yourself on any level, you have lost the power of Crow. Think about it, and maybe your inner truth will come to you.

In seeing what is true, you may need to weed out past beliefs or ideas to bring yourself into the present moment. Contrary Crow speaks of needing to remember that Divine Law is *not* judgment or denial of self-truths. Divine Law is honoring harmony that comes from a peaceful mind, an open heart, a true tongue, a light step, a forgiving nature, and a love of all living creatures. Honor the past as your teacher, honor the present as your creation, and honor the future as your inspiration.

Refusing to honor the shifts in your reality can cause emotional pain. An implosion of energy is apparent when rebellion surfaces. Contrary Crow speaks of broken law. The law of expansion is broken by suppression. This may apply to a situation, an old habit, a person you have given your authority to, or your own fears. It is always your own creation, so call on Crow and shift that creation to your new reality.

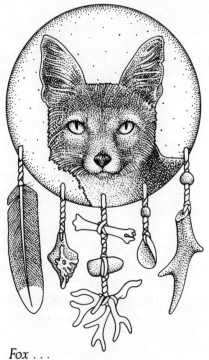

Fox . . .

    Where are you?
       Under the ferns?
          Becoming the forest,
            So I can learn?

Are you watching,
    Invisible to me?

        Trying to teach me,
          To become a tree?

25
Fox

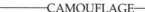

---CAMOUFLAGE---

Wily Fox has many allies in the woodlands, including the foliage, which offers protection and much medicine. Fox is seemingly able to vanish amidst the lush undergrowth of the forest. This flora is Fox's ally. The ability to meld into one's surroundings and be unnoticed is a powerful gift when one is observing the activities of others.

Another natural gift of Fox is the ability to adapt to winter by changing color, like the chameleon. Its rich, white, winter coat allows Fox to blend into the snow when the leaves no longer linger. Fox medicine involves adaptability, cunning, observation, integration, and swiftness of thought and action. These traits may also include quick decisiveness, and sure-footedness in the physical world.

Fox's ability to be unseen allows it to be the protector of the family unit. If danger arises, Fox is johnny-on-the-spot. Nanih Waiya, Great Spirit in the Choctaw tongue, honors Fox with the duty of keeping the family together and safe. This is accomplished through Fox's ability to observe undetected, without making others self-conscious. Fox is always concerned with the safety of family members and is an excellent talisman for those traveling far afield.

If Fox has chosen to share its medicine with you, it is a sign that you are to become like the wind, which is unseen yet is able to weave into and through any location or situation. You would be wise to observe the acts of others rather than their words at this time. Use your cunning nature in a positive way; keep silent about who and what and why you are observing. In learning the art of camouflage, you need to test your abilities to pull this off.

One test or exercise that may be helpful to you is deciding to be invisible. In doing this exercise, you might try to visualize your body as part of your surroundings, full of the colors of the location you are in. See yourself in your mind's eye, moving with stealth and grace, unheeded by others. If you do it right, it works! You can leave a party unnoticed or become as unobtrusive as a piece of furniture, watching the developing drama of the subjects you are studying.

While learning from Fox, you might also gain confidence in your ability to know instantly what will happen next. After observing for a while, you will become aware of a certain predictability in given situations and be able to quickly make your move. Fox medicine teaches the art of Oneness through its understanding of camouflage. This applies on all levels, from rocks to God. With Fox medicine, you are being asked to see all types of uses for Oneness.

Much like the clowns at the rodeo, Fox can keep the raging bull from stampeding a friend or family member. Fox can use silly tactics as a brilliant camouflage move. No one could guess the sly power behind such ingenious maneuvers.

CONTRARY:

Watch out for wily Fox if this card has appeared reversed! Someone may be watching you, and trying to figure out your next move. If you look deeper, however, it may be that you are watching yourself to *prove* to yourself that you exist. If you have become a "wallflower" to the point of disappearing, you may need to decide that you are worth noticing.

Contrary Fox is as foolish as it is cunning, and you may have fooled yourself into believing that your low self-esteem is due to your being born plain or having an ordinary life. This is camouflage of a different sort, in that you have camouflaged your true desire to experience life with friends, with joy, and with purpose. In any case, you are put on notice to be aware of apathy and self-induced boredom. You may have to dig deeply to find what excites you enough to scurry across the wasteland of your dulled senses and *live*.

Contrary Fox may also be telling you that you have become *too* visible. In climbing to a place of recognition, oftentimes the envy or jealousness of others is thrown in your face. If you are feeling attacked, withdraw. It may be time to assume the attitude of the hermit and deck yourself in the cloak of invisibility.

To right contrary Fox in this situation, call on Armadillo and name your boundaries. Then call on the family's protector to show you the art of camouflage. Once out of the line of attack, you can resume the role of being your "foxy" self.

Become Fox and feel the joy of knowing the playground of your life. You may just find the chicken coop full of intriguing morsels of delight.

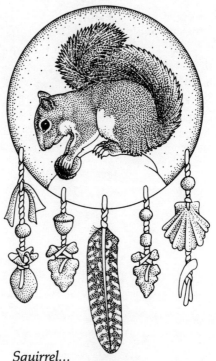

Squirrel...
   You have gathered
      Nuts by the score,
  Exactly predicting
      If you'll need more.

Teach me to take
     No more than I need.
Trusting Great Mystery
      To harvest the seed.

26
Squirrel

---GATHERING---

Squirrel teaches you to plan ahead for the winter when the trees are bare and the nuts have long since disappeared. Squirrel medicine can come in many forms, as this furry creature is very diverse in nature. The erratic behavior of Squirrel has bested many a forlorn hunter, and it thus stands to reason that there are benefits to being able to circle a branch at lightning speed. This erratic behavior of Squirrel can also get nerve-wracking if you are dealing with persons who have Squirrel medicine. Trying to calm them down enough to accomplish something may drive you nuts!

The gathering power of Squirrel medicine is a great gift. It teaches you how to gather and store your energy for times of need. It teaches you to reserve something for future use, whether it be a judgment, an opinion, a savings account, candles, or extra food. To put it in a nutshell, Squirrel is the Boy Scout of the animal kingdom—always prepared.

In today's world of changing times and fortunes, it is the wise person who prepares for the future. Our prophesies have all spoken of the end of the millennium and the changes to come. Squirrel is a friendly medicine to have, in light of possible future rainy days. Its message is to be prepared, but not to go nuts with it. Love yourself enough to gather the goods that will meet your needs in times of scarcity, even if that time never comes.

If Squirrel has scurried into your cards today, it may be that you are being told to honor your future by readying yourself for change. The message could be to lighten your load if you have gathered too many "things" that do *not* serve you. These "things" can include thoughts, worries, pressures, stresses, or gadgets that have been broken for years. In understanding the balance involved in gathering, you need to look at the idea of circulating the stock of what you have gathered. Call the nearest thrift store and give the gadgets to someone who can benefit from them. If something no longer "grows corn" for you, then it is time to let it go.

Squirrel has another lesson which can aid you if you observe what is obvious, and which can prepare you for anything. It has to do with the safe place in which to put your gatherings. This safe place is an untroubled heart and mind, and that which is gathered to put in this place is wisdom and caring. The energies gathered will set your mind and heart free, so that you will know that all will be taken care of in its own time. Apply this to your fears about the future and they will vanish.

CONTRARY:

The contrary medicine of Squirrel is the hoarder: a fearful person who expects the worst and is stuck in waiting. Waiting for something to happen is the trap. No action equals stagnation, but a little of Squirrel's erratic energy might get things moving. If Squirrel is hanging upside down on your branch, you may have begun seeing the world through opposites, hoarding your thoughts of abundance so that fear of scarcity takes hold. You may ask yourself:

1) Have I denied my ability to produce enough space for abundance to enter my life?

2) Have I denied my connection to the Earth Mother, from whom all things flow?

3) In moving too fast, have I taken on the erratic nature of Squirrel without having any focus?

4) Am I leaking my energy on worry instead of gathering power through being prepared?

Remember, one of the Squirrel family gathered the energy of Eagle and connected to the Great Spirit . . . now this Squirrel can fly.

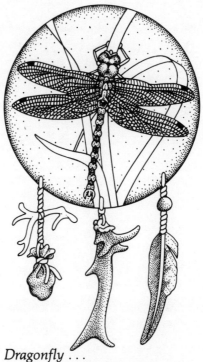

Dragonfly . . .
  Breaks illusions,
    Brings visions of power,
      No need to prove it,
        Now is the hour!

  Know it, believe it,
    Great Spirit intercedes,

  Feeding you, blessing you,
    Filling all your needs.

27
Dragonfly

---ILLUSION---

Dragonfly medicine is of the dreamtime and the illusionary facade we accept as physical reality. The iridescence of Dragonfly's wings reminds us of colors not found in our everyday experience. Dragonfly's shifting of color, energy, form, and movement explodes into the mind of the observer, bringing vague memories of a time or place where magic reigned.

Some legends say that Dragonfly was once Dragon, and that Dragon had scales like Dragonfly's wings. Dragon was full of wisdom, and flew through the night bringing light with its fiery breath. The breath of Dragon brought forth the art of magic and the illusion of changing form. Then Dragon got caught in its own facade. Coyote tricked Dragon into changing form, and the shape of its new body became like Dragonfly's. In accepting the challenge to prove its power and magical prowess, Dragon lost its power.

Dragonfly is the essence of the winds of change, the messages of wisdom and enlightenment, and the communications from the elemental world. This elemental world is made up of the tiny spirits of plants, and of the elements air, earth, fire, and water. In essence, this world is full of nature spirits.

If Dragonfly has flown into your cards today, you may have forgotten to water your plants. On another level, you may need to give thanks to the foods you eat for sustaining your body. On the psychological level, it may be time to break down the illusions you have held that restrict your actions or ideas.

Dragonfly medicine always beckons you to seek out the parts of your habits which you need to change. Have you put on too much weight, or have you started to look like a scarecrow? Have you tended to the changes you have wanted to make in your life? If you feel the need for change, call on Dragonfly to guide you through the mists of illusion to the pathway of transformation.

See how you can apply the art of illusion to your present question or situation, and remember that things are never completely as they seem.

CONTRARY:

Are you trying to prove to yourself or someone else that you have power? Are you caught in an illusion that weakens your true feelings or minimizes your abilities? If so, you may have contracted "Dragonfly dive-bombing." Is this the final "crash and burn" for some pipe dream that had no real purpose? Look within and feel the sense-of-self energy within yourself. Notice if it is ebbing, and find the point in time when you were deluded into believing that you would be happier if you changed because someone else wanted you to. Misery is a prime clue that you lost your will and personal validity when you bought into someone else's idea of who or what you should be. The *illusion* was that you would be happier if you did it their way. In forfeiting what you know is right and true for you personally, you give away your power. It is time for you to take it back.

Follow Dragonfly to the place inside your body where magic is still alive, and drink deeply of its power. This strength belongs to you. It is the power of becoming the illusion. This ability is ever changing, and contains within it the knowledge that *you are creating it all*.

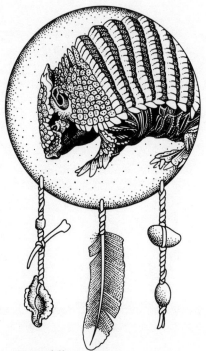

Armadillo . . .

Armor all my boundaries,
Teach me my shields,
Reflect all the hurt,
So I will not yield.

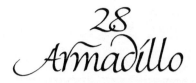

28
Armadillo

---BOUNDARIES---

Armadillo wears its armor on its back, its medicine a part
of its body. Its boundaries of safety are a part of its total being.
Armadillo can roll into a ball and never be penetrated
by enemies.

What a gift it is to set your boundaries so that harmful words
or intentions just roll off. Your lesson is in setting up what you
are willing to experience. If you do not wish to experience
feeling invaded, just call on Armadillo medicine.

A clue to how to proceed is to make a circle on a piece of
paper and see it as a medicine shield. In the body of the shield,
write all that you are desiring to have, do, or experience. Include
all things that give you joy. This sets up boundaries that allow
only these chosen experiences to be a part of your life. These
boundaries become a shield that wards off the things which are
undesirable to you. The shield reflects *what* you are and what
your will is to others on an unconscious level. Outside of the
shield you may put what you are willing to experience "by
invitation only," for example a visit from a long lost relative,
or criticism from friends, or people needing handouts.

If Armadillo has waddled into the cards you chose, it is
time to define your space. You may have been too willing to let
your home become a bus station. You may find that you cannot
say "no" even when you know that you will have to cancel
plans to be obliging. This routine can get old in a hurry!

It may be time to ask yourself the following questions:

1) Am I honoring the time I need for my personal enjoyment?

2) Do others treat me like a doormat?

3) Why do I always get upset when I'm taken for granted?

4) Is there a reason for my being a "yes" person?

All of the answers to these questions relate to setting up boundaries: what you will and won't do; what makes you feel uncomfortable and what is comforting to you. How you react in any circumstance has to do with your ability to be objective. You cannot be objective if you cannot tell where the other person's personality stops and where yours begins. If you have no boundaries, you are like a sponge. It will seem as if all the feelings in a room full of people *must be yours*. Ask yourself if you are really feeling depressed, or if this feeling actually belongs to the person you are talking to. Then allow Armadillo's armor to slice in-between, giving you back your sense of self.

CONTRARY:

Go ahead, roll up and hide. This, sarcastically, is the message of reversed Armadillo. You may think the only way to win in your present situation is to hide or to pretend that you are armor-coated and invincible, but this is not the way to grow. It is better to open up and find the value and strength of your vulnerability. You will experience something wonderful if you do.

Vulnerability is the key to enjoying the gifts of physical life. In allowing yourself to feel, a myriad of expressions are made available. For instance, a true compliment is an admiration flow of energy. If you are afraid of being hurt and are hiding from feeling anything, you will never feel the joy of admiration from others.

The key is in allowing Armadillo to help you to stop hiding, and to use Armadillo's armor to deflect negative energies. In this way you are able to accept or reject any feeling, action, or energy flow without having to hide from it.

The underside of Armadillo is soft, but its armor will protect this softness if the boundaries are in place. Hiding from your true feelings and fearing failure or rejection will *amplify* your need for cast-iron protection. You have the power to rid yourself of these doubts and to touch the deepest part of beingness. You will know you are doing the right thing. Whether it is communicating, or painting, or surfing — the creation belongs to you.

The only real rejection is in not trying to break out of the armor you have used to protect yourself. Is the armor now becoming a jail, and your fears the jailer?

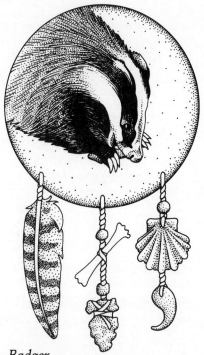

Badger ...
   Badger ...
      Badger ...

Until you reach your goal,
   Know the inner power,
      That lives in your soul.

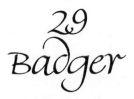

29
Badger

---------------AGGRESSIVENESS---------------

Badger is vicious, and attacks with powerful aggression. Badger is quick to anger and quicker to pounce. The power of Badger's medicine is aggressiveness and the willingness to fight for what it wants.

The very thought of facing Badger makes other animals run for cover. Like Skunk, Badger's reputation precedes it. Its hissing fangs will tear less aggressive opponents to shreds.

Badger is the medicine of many powerful medicine women, for Badger is also the keeper of the medicine roots. Badger sees all the roots of Mother Earth's healing herbs hanging in its burrow home. These roots are a key to aggressive healing.

Roots can ground negative energy into the Earth by allowing illness to pass through a body into the ground as neutral energy. Badger medicine people are quick to act in a crisis, and they do not panic.

If Badger is a part of your medicine, you are quick to express your feelings, and you do not care what the consequences are. Badger people oftentimes insist on carrying the ball for the touchdown. This attitude, however, does not endear them to their teammates.

Badger medicine may also point to the aggressive healer who will have the courage to use unconventional means to exact a cure. Like the mother who sits for days nursing a child with high fever, Badger is willing to persist.

Badger people can be vicious gossips, or may exhibit a "chip on the shoulder" syndrome if they are out of balance. You can be sure that people with Badger medicine will be aggressive enough to make it to the tops of their chosen fields, because they do not give up. They are also the finest healers, because they will use any and all methods to ensure healing, and will not give up on the critically ill.

A Badger person is often the "boss," and the one that everyone fears. That same boss will surely keep any company afloat. Badger gets the job accomplished. Badger's certainty is a source of strength.

If Badger pushed its way into your cards today, it may be telling you that you have been too meek in trying to reach some goal. Badger asks you how long you are willing to sit and wait for the world to deliver your silver spoon.

In this medicine, the key is to become aggressive enough to *do* something about your present state of affairs. Badger is teaching you to get angry in a creative way and say, "I won't take it anymore." You must follow-up by keeping your eye on the goal. Honor the healing process as you express those inner feelings.

Be aggressive, but don't cut others to ribbons on the way — that is too much aggression. Use your anger to stop your lolling around, so that your doldrums of apathy are a thing of the past. Badger is a powerful medicine when properly used for self-improvement.

Remember that Badger may be signalling a time when you can use your healing abilities to push ahead in life. Heal yourself by aggressively removing the barriers that don't "grow corn." Cut away the dead wood and use Badger's aggression to seek new levels of expression. Use Badger's medicine roots to keep grounded and centered in the process.

CONTRARY:

Oops! Here comes Badger upside-down and fuming! This could mean that you are being chewed out by someone else, or that you have expressed your anger in an unhealthy way. If this applies to you, remember that *all anger* stems from anger toward the self. It is an anger of helplessness that is misdirected toward others.

If you are angry at a coworker for telling the boss that you were looking for another job, you are really angry at yourself for not keeping your own secret. If you are angry at your children for disobeying, it is usually anger that stems from *fear* for the children's well-being. This self-anger condition is usually present when you have "silly accidents," falls, cuts and scrapes, or when you find yourself bumping into furniture.

Badger in the contrary position can issue in a time of reflection on what you feel helpless about. Is it your lack of aggressiveness or initiative? Is it your fear of being blasted or belittled if you present a new idea? Maybe it is a time when you need to get in touch with your own jealousy or envy of others who are willing to put themselves on top through hard work.

In the reverse, Badger teaches you the pitfalls of shyness and insecurity as well as of misused or vicious aggression. Go to your feelings — maybe you just need to let off steam. If so, scream into a pillow and then punch it a few times. It will surely put Badger back into balance. Badger can be difficult medicine, and learning to use it properly is a rare gift.

In another context, contrary Badger could be calling you to use herbs and roots to heal your body. Badger reversed may also be putting you on notice to be aware of those areas of your life that need the input of someone else's aggressive creativity to spark your own. In any case, contrary Badger speaks of a need for more aggressive action in life. No more inactivity can prevail without creating pain of some kind.

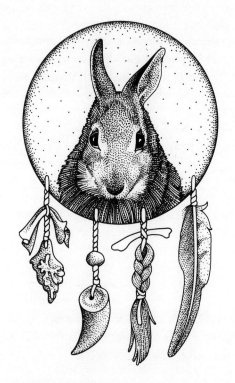

Scared little Rabbit . . .
   Please drop your fright!
      Running doesn't stop the pain,
         Or turn the dark to light.

30
Rabbit

---FEAR---

A long time ago — no one really knows how long ago it was — Rabbit was a brave and fearless warrior. Rabbit was befriended by Eye Walker, a witch. The witch and Rabbit spent much time together sharing and talking. The two were very close.

One day Eye Walker and Rabbit were walking along and they sat down on the trail to rest. Rabbit said, "I'm thirsty." Eye Walker picked up a leaf, blew on it, and then handed Rabbit a gourd of water. Rabbit drank the water but didn't say anything. Then Rabbit said, "I'm hungry." Eye Walker picked up a stone and blew on it and changed it to a turnip. She gave the turnip to Rabbit to eat. Rabbit tasted it and then ate the turnip with relish. But still Rabbit didn't say anything.

The two continued along the trail, which led into the mountains. Near the top, Rabbit tripped and fell and rolled almost to the bottom. Rabbit was in very sad condition when Eye Walker got to him. She used a magic salve on Rabbit to heal his great pain and mend his broken bones. Rabbit didn't say anything.

Several days later Eye Walker went searching for her friend. She searched high and low but Rabbit was nowhere to be found.

Finally, Eye Walker gave up. She met Rabbit quite by accident one day. "Rabbit, why are you hiding and avoiding me?" the witch asked.

"Because I am afraid of you. I am afraid of magic," answered Rabbit, cowering. "Leave me alone!"

"I see," said Eye Walker. "I have used my magical powers on your behalf and now you turn on me and refuse my friendship."

"I want nothing more to do with you or your powers," Rabbit countered. Rabbit did not even see the tears his words were bringing to Eye Walker's eyes. "I hope we never meet and that I never see you again," Rabbit continued.

"Rabbit," Eye Walker said, "We once were great friends and companions, but no more. It is within my power to destroy you, but because of the past and the medicines we have shared together I will not do this. But from this day forward I lay a curse on you and your tribe. From now on, you will call your fears and your fears will come to you. Be on your way, for the sweet medicines that bound us together as friends are broken."

Now Rabbit is the Fear Caller. He goes out and shouts, "Eagle, I am so afraid of you." If Eagle doesn't hear him, Rabbit calls louder, "Eagle, stay away from me!" Eagle, now hearing Rabbit, comes and eats him. Rabbit calls bobcats, wolves, coyotes, and even snakes until they come.

As this story shows, Rabbit medicine people are so afraid of tragedy, illness, disaster, and "being taken," that they call those very fears to them to teach them lessons. The keynote here is: what you resist will persist! What you fear most is what you will become.

Here is the lesson. If you pulled Rabbit, stop talking about horrible things happening and get rid of "what if" in your vocabulary. This card may signal a time of worry about the future or of trying to exercise your control over that which is not yet in form — the future. *Stop now!* Write your fears down and be willing to feel them. Breathe into them, and feel them running through your body into Mother Earth as a give-away.

CONTRARY:

The paralyzed feeling which Rabbit experiences when being stalked is Rabbit in the contrary position. If you have tried to resolve a situation in your life and are unable to, you may be feeling frozen in motion. This could indicate a time to wait for the forces of the universe to start moving again. It could also indicate the need to stop and take a rest. It will always indicate a time when you need to re-evaluate the process you are undergoing, and to rid yourself of any negative feelings, barriers, or duress. Simply put, you cannot have your influence felt until you rearrange your way of seeing the present set of circumstances.

There is always a way out of any situation, because the Universal Force does move on. It is the way in which you handle problems that allows you to succeed.

Take a hint from Rabbit. Burrow into a safe space to nurture yourself and release your fears until it is time again to move into the pasture, clear of prowlers who want a piece of your juicy energy.

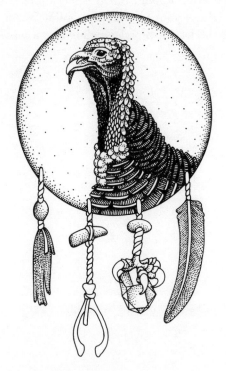

Ho, Brother Turkey!
So freely you give,
Of everything that you are,
So others may truly live.

31
Turkey

---------------GIVE-AWAY---------------

Turkey is actually thought to be the Give-Away Eagle or
South Eagle of many Native peoples. The philosophy of give-
away was practiced by many tribes. Simply stated, it is the
deep and abiding recognition of the sacrifices of both self and
others. People in modern-day society, who have many times
more than they need, should study the noble turkey who sacrifices itself so that we may live. In Turkey's death we have our
life. Honor Turkey.

Spectators unfamiliar with the cultural phenomenon of the pot-
latch or give-away ceremony are often mystified by it. A tribal
member may gladly give away all he or she owns, and do without
in order to help the People. In present-day urban life, we are taught
to acquire and get ahead. The person with the most toys wins the
game. In some cultures, no one can win the game unless *the whole*
of the People's needs are met. A person who claims more than his
or her share is looked upon as selfish or crazy or both. The poor,
the aged, and the feeble have honor. The person who gives away
the most and carries the burdens of the People is one of the most
respected.

Turkey was the medicine of many saints and mystics. Celebrate
if you have Turkey medicine. Your virtues are many. You have
transcended self. You act and react on the behalf of others. You
aspire to help those who need help. This is not out of some
sense of self-righteous moralism or religious guilt. Help and
sustenance are given by Turkey out of the realization that all
life is sacred. It is knowing that the Great Spirit resides within
all people. It is an acknowledgement that what you do for
others you do for yourself. Turkey medicine rests in true ego,
in enlightenment. Doing unto others and feeding the People

is the message of all true spiritual systems.

Depending on how Turkey is aspected in your cards, you are being given a gift. This gift could be spiritual, material, or even intellectual. The gift may be great or small, but it is never insignificant. Congratulations. You may have just won the lottery. Or the gift may be a beautiful sunset, or the smell of a fragrant flower. On the other hand, you may feel the "spirit of giving" growing within you, and wanting you to share with others.

CONTRARY:

There are several aspects to pulling the gobbler card in the reversed position. Are you gobbling up anything and everything out of fear of lack? Are you holding on too tight and refusing to let go of a dime for charity? It could be that the Scrooge in you has grown accustomed to the miserly aspect of living. If not, you might look at the possibility that you are fearful of spending money at this time. Another aspect of "contrary gobbling" is the idea that the world "owes" you something and that you do not need to recycle the energy. "The buck stops here" may only mean that it stops in your bank account. On all levels of this contrary message, the keynote is that generosity of spirit is being neglected. This can be toward self or toward others.

Remember, never give to receive. That is manipulation. Giving is without regret and with a joyful heart, or the "give-away" has lost its true meaning.

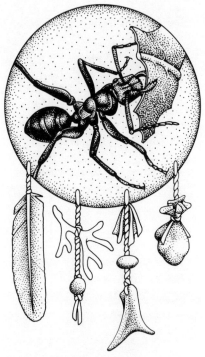

Oh tiny Ant . . .
   Your patience grows,
      Like the sands of time.

Can I learn to be like you?
   Or is it too sublime?

32
Ant

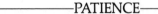

————————PATIENCE————————

Ant can carry a leaf over hundreds of miles just to get it back to the anthill. Ants in Africa will strip a forest bare when food is scarce, if it takes them a year. Ant's medicine is the strategy of patience. Ant is a builder like Beaver, is aggressive like Badger, has stamina like Elk, scrutiny like Mouse, and give-away like Turkey.

Every Ant in an anthill is part of the Ant "group mind," as all the Ants work for the Queen Ant and the hive. Self-sacrifice is a part of Ant medicine. Greater than Ant's other medicines, however, is patience.

Ant people are active, community-minded folks who see the greater future needs of their town. Ant people are planners, like Squirrel, and are content to see their dreams being built a little at a time. In today's society that is a rare quality.

In the desert, one type of Ant will burrow a conical hole with its apex at the bottom. The Ant will cover itself and patiently wait for some unsuspecting insect to fall in. As the sand crumbles, the prey eventually falls to the bottom, only to find Ant's open jaws.

Patience does have its rewards!

Ant people have a knowing about the sweet victory at the end of the line. There is never a concern about "going without" if they are late for the opening of a sale. If what they want is sold out, they are sure that something equal or better is available.

If you have Ant medicine, you eat slowly and deliberately and are content in knowing that "what is yours will come to you." This knowing is good medicine. It shows a trust in the Universe to provide.

If Ant meandered into your spread today, it is time to show a little trust and patience in some life situation. You may have forgotten that you will always receive that which you need, at the time you need it most. If it is not on the horizon or just around the next anthill, you may need to use some strategy. How can you put to use your power of creation until "it" arrives — whatever "it" means to you at this time?

Ant is working for the good of the whole. Are you? If you are, be assured that the whole wants the same goodness for you, and that it will be provided.

CONTRARY:

Watch out! Here comes the sting! If you are in a hurry, you may fall prey to those who are not working for the good of the whole of humanity. Those individuals who make greed a way of life prey on the fear and urgency of those who have forgotten natural and tribal law. It's easy money! If this warning applies to you, become aware of users and con artists.

In the contrary position, Ant also teaches you to *trust* natural law. If you do, harmony always follows. Your silly impatience will bring Coyote to aid you in sabotaging your plans for the future if you allow your panic to outweigh your rational sensibilities. The key here is to honor the will of the Great Spirit, so that mountains are not made out of anthills!

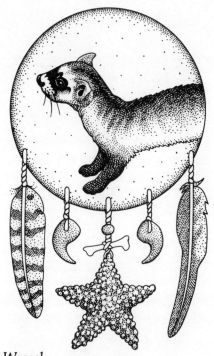

Weasel . . .
    Weasel . . .
        Weasel . . .

Who's in the hen house now?
    If I were to ask you,
        You'd say it was the Cow!!

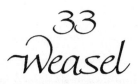

33
Weasel

---STEALTH---

Weasel has an incredible amount of energy and ingenuity, yet it is a difficult power totem to have. It is not without significance that ermine or weasel pelt is worn by royalty. Weasel ears hear what is really being said. This is a great ability. Weasel eyes see beneath the surface of a situation to know the many ramifications of an event. This too is a rare gift.

The chiefs sent Weasel to the enemy camp to smoke them for power. "What are the medicines of the enemy?" the chiefs asked Weasel upon its return.

Weasel never failed to give an accurate account of the enemy's numbers, strengths, and weaknesses. It was Weasel who tearfully told the Original People of the coming of the white boat people. "These brothers have strange new medicines," said Weasel. "They will tell us that to live the way we do is wrong. They will confuse us with their talking bark. They have stolen thunder from Sky Father and placed it in their weapons. They have no respect for the animal brothers and sisters, and they make their thunder speak to the animals and kill them. They will make the thunder speak to us also. Their numbers are too many to count, and these white brothers will steal everything from us but our spirits. The great dark shadow of the ravenous bird of death has fallen over the People."

Weasel fur changes color with the season. Silent Weasel has many lessons to teach you. Weasel could confound Great Spirit, pick Great Spirit's pockets, and then leave Great Spirit contemplating the divine navel. If this is your personal medicine, your powers of observation are keen. You seem to be saying, "Leave me alone and I will do the same for you." You might even look a bit guilty at times due to what you know from observing life.

You may be a loner hiding yourself away from others, or perhaps even a recluse. You are a powerful ally to have in any business organization since you can see what the competition is doing. People may make a great mistake in sizing you up since they do not immediately see your powers. But the first time they try to outsmart you, they will soon learn that your intelligence is greater than their own.

Look to Weasel power to tell you the "hidden reasons" behind anything. Some people are put off by Weasel medicine, talent, and abilities, but there are no bad medicines. We all have power, or we would not be here to heal Mother Earth. Perhaps if you have Weasel power you could use your secret gifts for the good of all. Observe who or what needs attention, or a solution, and offer your assistance in your own quiet or discreet way.

CONTRARY:

Is contrary Weasel in your cards? If so, look out for intrigue. Someone may be using covert tactics to Weasel into the hen house. Perhaps you should lock your doors and dress your teenager like a nun. Or perhaps you may be lying to yourself about something you know to be true. This can be a lie on any level, for instance, storming the refrigerator at 3:00 A.M. and telling yourself no one will miss the half-eaten portion of the pie. If you scratch someone else's automobile in a parking lot, leave a note. Don't slink away just because you can. Honesty to self and others is of the utmost importance.

Another message of reversed Weasel is to acknowledge why you have been doubting your feelings. Weasel upright observes all actions, feelings, and situations with keen senses. In the contrary, those abilities of observation are dulled until confusion sets in. When you don't know how you feel or what is occurring around you, doubt becomes the barrier to your progress. Then you may find a bit of paranoia seeping into your life.

If you want to right the situation, start by shaking the dullness out of your head and observing the obvious. No one can fool you if you watch your step, honor your knowing, seek the "hidden reasons," and use discretion in the process.

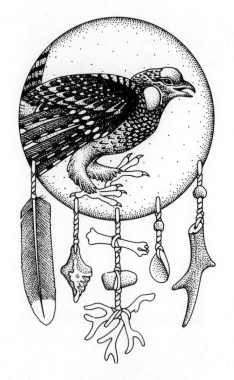

Grouse . . . of the Sacred Spiral,
   Leading us on,
      To reach the everlasting heights,

Where we can live as one.

34
Grouse

-SACRED SPIRAL-

Grouse once flocked in abundance throughout North America, but now, even on the plains where these birds were so plentiful, there is an absence of them. Many Plains Indian tribes dance the Grouse Dance to honor these birds. The movement of the dance follows a spiral, which is the ancient symbol of birth and rebirth, the ribbed tunnel of eternal return.

The Sacred Spiral is also one of the oldest known symbols for personal power. When you think of Grouse medicine, visualize a whirlpool or even a tornado, for the Sacred Spiral will take you to the center. The spiral is a metaphor for personal vision and enlightenment. Many initiates on Vision Quests paint spirals on their bodies and believe that the Great Mystery will favor them with visions of power and purpose because of this symbol.

The whirling dervishes of certain Sufi orders are masters of the spiral dance and can transcend to higher states of awareness through the repetition of this sacred movement. It is said that dervishes can travel to the center of the spiral and return with any magical power they choose. In the dervish state, one enters the Great Silence and has direct communication with the Creator By spinning clockwise or counter-clockwise, the dervish draws or repulses specific energies. Sufi dancing is a system which connects one with the Divine Source through ritual treatment of motion.

If you have Grouse medicine in your cards, undertake a meditation on the various qualities of movement within your world. Begin by visualizing the Sun as one member of a huge group of stars swirling in the massive pinwheel shape of the Milky Way. Then draw yourself out of this pinwheel of light and into the spiralling of your own DNA's double helix, an arrangement similar to a rope ladder coiled like a corkscrew.

Analyze the way you move through your world. How do you picture yourself in the act of "locomotion?" What kind of reaction do you create with the energy you send into the universe? What words would you use to describe the way you move through both the material and spiritual worlds? In the final analysis, is your movement compatible with your greatest desires and goals?

Many spiritual disciplines ask that you cease all external movement in order to recognize the inner life. Grouse medicine, however, is an invitation to the dance. Grouse celebrates the Divine Source through its sacred spiral dance, and offers *this dance* to you as a gift. You can spend a lifetime learning Grouse's lesson on how to harmonize your dance with Mother Earth's cycles, and how to offer the dance as a creation of selfless beauty.

CONTRARY:

Drawing the Grouse medicine card in the reverse position signals a dissipation of energy and lack of control and discipline. It is symbolic of a lost connection to the Source, and signifies a lack of clear intent behind an outpouring of energy. You may feel like you are in a tailspin or going down the drain. Confront confusion either in yourself or in others who may be in the picture. Examine the way your energy may be causing friction, sparks, or a convolution of a situation that needs clarification. Work toward harnessing your energy and directing it toward clearly defined goals. Such is the nature of the Sacred Grouse Dance.

In using this sacred dance as a tool to right contrary Grouse, you may also find that it is a tool to center or ground you. In grounding, you are once again connecting to Mother Earth and balancing out the spinning in your head. If you have become so involved with an idea or problem that you are no longer seeing it clearly, you may feel dizzy or lacking in concentration. This is a sign that you have entered the thought-universe and are not connected to physical reality. You need grounding if this occurs.

Dancing or walking will put you back in touch with Earth and your body. Grouse may then teach you how to notice the energy flows that put you in harmony and balance with body, mind, and spirit.

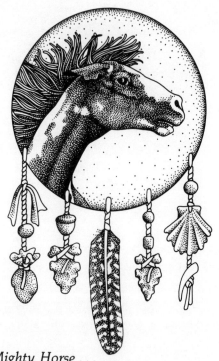

Mighty Horse . . .
   Power to run
      Across the open plains,

Or to bring the vision,
   Of the shields
      Dancing in purple dream rain.

35
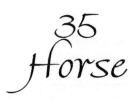
Horse

---POWER---

"Stealing horses is stealing power" was a statement made frequently in historical Native America and a reference to the esteemed role which Horse played in the Native cultures.

Horse is physical power *and* unearthly power. In shamanic practices throughout the world, Horse enables shamans to fly through the air and reach heaven.

Humanity made a great leap forward when Horse was domesticated, a discovery akin to that of fire. Before Horse, humans were earthbound, heavy-laden, and slow creatures indeed. Once humans climbed on Horse's back, they were as free and fleet as the wind. They could carry burdens for great distances with ease. Through their special relationship with Horse, humans altered their self-concept beyond measure. Horse was the first animal medicine of civilization. Humanity owes an incalculable debt to Horse and to the new medicine it brought. It would be a long walk to see one's brother or sister if Horse had not welcomed the two-legged rider upon its back. Today we measure the capacity of engines with the term "horsepower," a reminder of the days when Horse was an honored and highly-prized partner with humanity.

Dreamwalker, a medicine man, was walking across the plains to visit the Arapaho Nation. He carried with him his pipe. The feather tied into his long black hair pointed to the ground, marking him as a man of peace. Over the rise of a hill, Dreamwalker saw a herd of wild mustangs running toward him.

Black Stallion approached him and asked if he was seeking an answer on his journey. Black Stallion said, "I am from the Void where Answer lives. Ride on my back and know the power of entering the Darkness and finding the Light." Dreamwalker thanked Black Stallion and agreed to visit him when his medicine was needed in the Dreamtime.

Yellow Stallion approached Dreamwalker next and offered to take him to the East, where illumination lives. Dreamwalker could share the answers he found there to teach and illuminate others. Once again, Dreamwalker thanked Yellow Stallion and said he would use these gifts of power on his journey.

Red Stallion approached, rearing playfully. He told Dreamwalker of the joys of balancing work and heavy medicine with the joyful experiences of play. He reminded Dreamwalker that he could better hold the attention of those he taught when humor was integrated with the lesson. Dreamwalker thanked him and promised to remember the gift of joy.

Dreamwalker was nearing his destination. The Arapaho Nation was close at hand. White Stallion came to the front of the herd. Dreamwalker mounted White Stallion's back. White Stallion was the message carrier for all the other horses, and represented wisdom in power. This magnificent horse was the embodiment of the balanced medicine shield. "No abuse of power will ever lead to wisdom," said White Stallion. "You, Dreamwalker, have made this journey to heal a brother in need, to share the sacred pipe, and to heal the Mother Earth. You have the knowledge through humility that you are an instrument of Great Spirit. As I carry you upon my back, you carry the needs of the people on yours. In wisdom, you understand that power is not given lightly but awarded to those who are willing to carry responsibility in a balanced manner."

Dreamwalker, the shaman, had been healed by the visit of the wild horses, and knew that his purpose in coming to the Arapaho was to share these gifts with them.

In understanding the power of Horse, you may see how to strive for a balanced medicine shield. True power is wisdom found in remembering your total journey. Wisdom comes from remembering pathways you have walked in another person's moccasins. Compassion, caring, teaching, loving, and sharing your gifts, talents, and abilities are the gateways to power.

CONTRARY:

If your ego has gotten in the way, you may have failed to notice the lack of respect you have been receiving from others. You may, on the other hand, be struggling with others who are abusing their power. "Should I say something? Should I fight my desire to put them in their place?" you may be asking. Remember the times in your own life when you have fallen out of grace with Great Spirit, and then have compassion for the brothers or sisters who are now doing the same. If you are overpowering another or feeling overwhelmed, Horse medicine in both the dignified *and* contrary positions is a simple reminder of *how* to balance your shields.

In allowing all pathways to have equal validity, you will see the power and glory of the unified *family of humanity*. This is the gift of the Rainbow Warrior or Warrioress. The "I" has no place in this Whirling Rainbow that comes from the Great Mystery and is replaced by the universal "we." All colors of the rainbow and all pathways are honored as one.

Apply this knowledge and reclaim the power you have given away by forgetting to come from compassion. Untangle yourself from the present situation and understand that every human being must follow this pathway to power before galloping upon the winds of destiny.

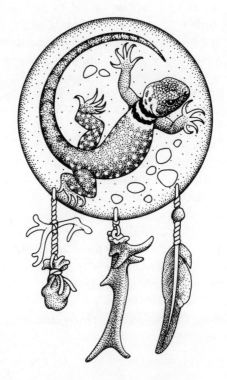

Lizard . . . will you dream with me?
Travel across the stars?
Beyond the place of time and space,
There live visions from afar.

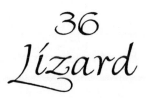

36
Lizard

---DREAMING---

Lizard sat lolling in the shadow of a big rock, shading himself from the desert sun. Snake crawled by, looking for some shadow to coil up in and rest. Snake watched Lizard for awhile as Lizard's eyeballs went side to side behind his enormous closed lids. Snake hissed to get Lizard's attention. Slowly Lizard's dreaming eyes opened and he saw Snake.

"Snake! You scared me! What do you want?" Lizard cried.

Snake spit his answer from his forked tongue. "Lizard, you are always getting the best shadow spots in the heat of the day. This is the only big rock for miles. Why don't you share your shade with me?"

Lizard thought for a moment, then agreed. "Snake, you can share my shade spot, but you have to go to the other side of the rock and you must promise not to interrupt me."

Snake was getting annoyed. He hissed, "How could I bother you, Lizard? All you are doing is sleeping."

Lizard smiled knowingly. "Oh Snake, you are such a silly serpent. I'm not sleeping. I'm dreaming."

Snake wanted to know what the difference was, so Lizard explained. "Dreaming is going into the future, Snake. I go to where *future* lives. You see, that is why I know you won't eat me today. I dreamed you and I know you're full of mouse."

Snake was taken aback. "Why Lizard, you're exactly right. I wondered why you said you would share your rock."

Lizard laughed to himself. "Snake," he said, "you are looking for shade and I am looking for shadow. Shadow is where the dreams live."

Lizard medicine is the shadow side of reality where your dreams are reviewed before you decide to manifest them physically.

Lizard could have created getting eaten by Snake if he had
so desired.

Lizard is the medicine of dreamers. Whether dreamers smoke
you or dream you, dreamers can always help you see the shadow.
This shadow can be your fears, your hopes, or the very thing
you are resisting, but it is always following you around like an
obedient dog.

If Lizard dreamed a space in your cards today, it may be
time to look and see what is following along behind you. Is it
your fears, your future trying to catch up to you, or is it the
part of you that wants to ignore your weaknesses and humanness?

Lizard may be telling you to pay attention to your dreams
and their symbols. Make a dream log and record all that you
remember. Be sure to pay attention to each individual symbol
or recurring pattern. If you do not remember your dreams, you
could try setting a music alarm for 2:00 a.m. or 3:00 a.m. Or
you could try drinking a lot of water before bedtime and allow
your bladder to wake you up. Dreams are very important. Pay
attention to them.

CONTRARY:

If Lizard has turned up in the contrary position, you may be
having a nightmare. This is a sign of inner conflict. Look to the
nightmare for a clue to the nature of this conflict. What are the
feelings your nightmare causes? Breathe through these feelings
and let the sensations flow out of your body. See the truth in
what your nightmare is suggesting. It could be the simple message
that you are confronting your fears and therefore do not need to
experience nightmarish events in your day-to-day life.

Another message of Lizard reversed is that you may need
more sleep or dreamtime. It could also imply that you have a
lack of dreams for your future.

Imagination is the door to all new ideas and creations. As
you examine the dreaming process, you will find that the sub-
conscious is processing *all* of the recorded messages it holds
concerning the events you experienced during the day. These
messages can be suppressed feelings bringing inner conflict, or

they can be new ideas or goals, other dimensions of awareness, future events, warning signals, or desires and hopes.

In one sense, contrary Lizard is insisting that you look to your imagination for new experience. This is necessary when life becomes dull or full of boredom. On the other hand, contrary Lizard may also apply to those who dream too much, refusing to use the dreams as *tools* to manifest that same vision in their lives.

All levels of awareness are accessible through dreams. Remember, life is not always as it seems. Are you the dreamer? Or are you the dreamed?

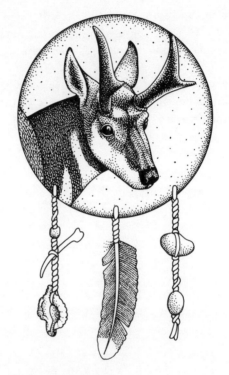

Run Antelope . . .
    Teach me,
        Of action
            And its pace.

Quickly,
    Quickly,
        So I may run with grace.

37
Antelope

---------ACTION---------

When time was just beginning and the "Tribe of Man" was small, Antelope saw that the two-leggeds were naked, hungry, and in danger of extinction. The Ancestors would soon vanish from Mother Earth if action were not taken.

Antelope took action and came into the camp, calling all the two-leggeds together for Council. "Great Mystery sent me to teach you a lesson. The lesson is to *do*. You have no need to be fearful if you know what to do and then you do it," Antelope said.

"And what shall we do?" asked the People.

"If you are naked and cold, you should kill me and take my coat to keep you warm. It is my gift to you. Do it."

"We will," said the People. "But what of our hunger. We are starving. What can we do to save ourselves?"

"If you are hungry, you should kill me and take my flesh, for it will nourish you and make you strong. It is my gift to you, and a part of my evolution. It is my service. Do it."

Antelope knew that humankind would survive the Ice Age if the People learned to eat meat. Before the movement of the great ice mountains, fruit and vegetables had been plentiful, and the two-leggeds had had no need to eat of the bodies of their fellow creatures. The clans of the second world ate Antelope. Taking the instinct and wisdom of the four-leggeds into their bodies, the People learned, through each creature's essence, how to survive. They were taught never to waste, or to take more than they needed. When they were in need, the two-leggeds knew to take action.

Humans learned Antelope's lesson well. Because of Antelope, humans took proper action and survived to this present day.

Antelope taught humans to honor the gifts sent from Great Mystery, and to avoid indiscriminate destruction of life.

Antelope signifies knowledgeable action. Antelope is a symbol for the antenna of your hair, which attaches you to Great Mystery by its long cords of light. Looking at Antelope, you become aware of your mortality and the short time span you have on this planet. With this in mind, you must act accordingly. Proper action pleases the Great Mystery. Antelope medicine is the knowledge of life's circle. Knowing of death, Antelope can truly live. Action is the key and essence of living.

Antelope powers have been courted and shamanized since the dawn of time. Antelope clans have been many, and the power of Antelope people is great. Antelope medicine gives you strength of mind and heart, and the ability to take quick and decisive action to get things accomplished.

If you feel stymied, call on Antelope medicine. If you are balled up and twisted in knots, Antelope powers will speak to you of proper action and soon set you free. Many ingenious solutions to problems are whispered by Antelope. Listen, and even more importantly, *act*. Surround yourself with the illumination and secret knowledge of Antelope. Combine this with action and you will overcome any obstacle or hindrance in your path. If Antelope is your Centering Tree and strong personal medicine, thank Great Spirit. Say what should be said. Your judgment is sound and your actions will be successful.

Always listen to what Antelope has to say to you. Antelope in your cards indicates a message of higher purpose. Antelope arms you with the Bow of Authority, and forces you to act on behalf of self, family, clan, nation, and finally Mother Earth. Antelope says, "Do it now. Don't wait any longer." Antelope knows the way, and so do you. Take courage and leap; your sense of timing is perfect. When Antelope has bounded into your cards, the time is *now*. The *power* is you.

CONTRARY:

Contrary Antelope is a signal that you are not listening, and not acting on the will of Great Spirit. You may be taking more than your share. Antelope medicine in the contrary makes you crazy and quarrelsome. You will certainly be indecisive and not know what direction to turn. You might be lying to yourself and others. Stop lying even if you think it will get you off the hook. Contrary Antelope will trip you at every turn. Quit being so conventional and following others all the time. Take your own authority. Let Antelope's heart beat strong in you, and you will know the way. But as always, the message is "Do it!" The fear of the unknown subsides once action begins.

Contrary Antelope may also be telling you that a *decision to start* is now necessary. The main element in procrastination is lack of conviction. To honor your *chosen* destiny is to honor your commitment to doing what you "proclaim" you are doing. Walking your talk is the essence of Antelope people. Talking your walk is contrary Antelope personified.

To right contrary Antelope, three steps are necessary:

1) Have the *desire* to do something.

2) Make the firm *decision* to begin that action.

3) Do it!

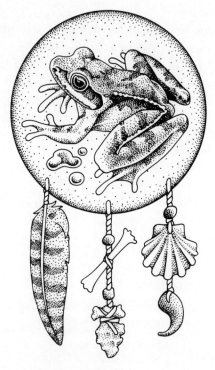

Sing Frog sing!
Call the rains,
   Quench the dryness,
    Cleanse the Earth,

Then fill me up again.

38
Frog

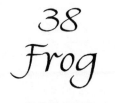

-------------------CLEANSING-------------------

Frog sings the songs that bring the rain and make the road dirt more bearable. Frog medicine is akin to water energy, and the East on the medicine wheel. Frog teaches us to honor our tears, for they cleanse the soul. All water rites belong to Frog, including all initiations by water.

Water prepares and cleanses the body for sacred ceremony. It is the element we understand best in the womb. Frog, like ourselves, is a pollywog in the fetal waters, and only learns to hop after it experiences the world of fluidity.

The transformation into adulthood prepares Frog for its power to call in the waters of the skies: The rain. In knowing the element of water, Frog can sing the song that calls the rain to Earth. When the ponds are dry, Frog calls upon the Thunder Beings to cleanse and replenish the Earth with water. Like Frog, we are asked to know when it is time to refresh, purify, and refill the coffers of the soul.

If Frog hopped into the cards you chose today, its "ribet" may be calling in the cleansing you need. If you were to look at where you are today, would you use any of the following words to describe your condition: tired, overloaded, harried, frustrated, guilty, itchy, nervous, at a loss, empty, or weakened?

If so, take a break and allow yourself to bathe in the waters of Frog medicine. This could mean a long, relaxing bath, disconnecting the phone, yelling "stop," or taking in deep, cleansing breaths.

The key thought is to find a way to rid yourself of distractions and to replace the mud with clear energy. Then replenish your parched spirit, body, and mind.

An ability of Frog medicine people is to give support and

energy where it is needed. A Frog medicine person can clean negativity from any environment. Many mediums or clairvoyants who work with cleaning "haunted" houses carry Frog medicine. Many of the world's seers use water on their hands when tapping into other realms of reality due to water's super-conductive nature.

In Mayan and Aztec shamanistic practices, the shaman places water in his or her mouth and sprays it over the body of a patient to clear away negative energy. This is done while holding the thought of Frog firmly in the mind so that healing may occur and the patient may be replenished with positive energy. Sometimes dried and stuffed Frogs are also used to guard the person's body during the session.

Frog speaks of new life and harmony through its rain song. The deep tones of Frog's "ribet" are said to be a call to the Thunder Beings: thunder, lightning, and rain. The "ribet" is the heartbeat that comes into harmony with Father Sky and calls for the replenishment needed. Call to Frog and find peace in the joy of taking time to give to yourself. A part of this giving is cleansing yourself of *any person, place, or thing* that does not contribute to your new state of serenity and replenishment.

CONTRARY:

Frog slipped in the mud and is lying on its back, unable to right itself. Get ready for more mud in your eye.

The contrary position of Frog can denote an unwillingness on your part to wipe the mire out of your life. Mud can turn from mire to bog to quicksand if you don't recognize its effect on your present situation.

Is someone draining your energy? Are you allowing yourself to ride down the tubes with them? Have you tried to settle someone else's quarrel and gotten in the line of fire? *Stop!* Recognize what it is that is mucking up the lily pond. Swim with Frog. Frog's bug eyes see it all. Dive deeply, and then hop to the next lily pad to catch the sun. In this way you may see exactly what has been draining your energy.

At times, all of life's activities can be overwhelming, and everyone occasionally needs a break. Contrary Frog can signal one of these moments, but can also portend a time of feeling waterlogged. In feeling waterlogged, you may be dealing with too many emotions or feelings. This is to say that "the world is too much with you," or that you have immersed yourself in one idea or activity to the exclusion of all other facets of your life. If this is the case, a break from routine is suggested. Hop to other lily pads or visit other ponds for awhile.

Negativity is drawn to you when you refuse to give yourself the time and space needed to assume a new viewpoint. Frog in the contrary position is an omen that you are courting disaster if you don't stop and smell the lilies, eat some flies, bask in the sun, and "ribet" until the rain comes to refill your spirit.

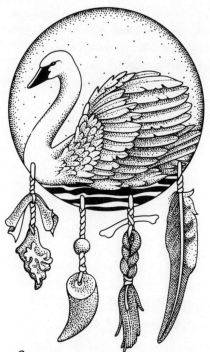

Swan . . .
　　The power of woman
　　　　Entering Sacred Space,

Touching future,
　　Yet to come,
　　　　Bringing eternal grace.

39
Swan

Little Swan flew through the Dreamtime, looking for the future. She rested for a moment in the coolness of the pond, looking for a way to find the entry point to the future. This was a moment of confusion for Swan, as she knew that she had happened into the Dreamtime by accident. This was her first flight alone and she was a bit concerned by the Dreamtime landscape.

As Swan looked high above Sacred Mountain, she saw the biggest swirling black hole she had ever seen. Dragonfly came flying by, and Swan stopped him to ask about the black hole. Dragonfly said, "Swan, that is the doorway to the other planes of imagination. I have been guardian of the illusion for many, many moons. If you want to enter there, you would have to ask permission and *earn* the right."

Swan was not so sure that she wanted to enter the black hole. She asked Dragonfly what was necessary for her to earn entry. Dragonfly replied, "You must be willing to accept whatever the future holds as it is presented, without trying to change Great Spirit's plan." Swan looked at her ugly little duckling body and then answered, "I will be happy to abide by Great Spirit's plan. I won't fight the currents of the black hole. I will *surrender* to the flow of the spiral and *trust* what I am shown." Dragonfly was very happy with Swan's answer and began to spin the magic to break the pond's illusion. Suddenly, Swan was engulfed by a whirlpool in the center of the pond.

Swan reappeared many days later, but now she was graceful and white and long-necked. Dragonfly was stunned! "Swan, what happened to you!" he exclaimed. Swan smiled and said, "Dragonfly, I learned to surrender my body to the power of

Great Spirit and was taken to where the future lives. I saw many wonders high on Sacred Mountain and because of my faith and my acceptance I have been changed. I have learned to accept the state of grace." Dragonfly was very happy for Swan.

Swan told Dragonfly many of the wonders beyond the illusion. Through her healing and her acceptance of the state of grace, she was given the right to enter the Dreamtime.

So it is that we learn to surrender to the grace of the rhythm of the universe, and slip from our physical bodies into the Dreamtime. Swan medicine teaches us to be at one with all planes of consciousness, and to trust in Great Spirit's protection.

If you pulled Swan, it ushers in a time of altered states of awareness and of development of your intuitive abilities. Swan medicine people have the ability to see the future, to surrender to the power of Great Spirit, and to accept the healing and transformation of their lives.

The Swan card is telling you to accept your ability to know what lies ahead. If you are resisting your self-transformation, relax; it will be easier if you go *with* the flow. Stop denying that you know who is calling when the phone rings. Pay attention to your hunches and your gut knowledge, and honor your female intuitive side.

CONTRARY:

If you have pulled Swan in reverse, it is a warning that you must acknowledge what you know, so stop denying your feelings and klutzing up. You may be bumping into furniture or forgetting what you are saying in mid-sentence. If so, this is a sign that you are not grounded. Jump in place and hold the top of your head as you do so. This will get you back in touch with the Earth, and keep you from wandering into a dreamy reality that lessens your focus. Baths help, as does going barefooted or doing some gardening.

In any case, Swan reversed says that you need to pay some attention to your body. It can seem as if you are flying without a pilot's license if you are not aware of when you take off or land. Not recognizing the shift from left brain to right brain is common when you are evolving spiritually. This is all a part of developing the intuitive side of your nature and is a sign that you are not being conscious of your entry into other levels of awareness. In the development of higher mind, you are embarking on new territory that has rules or universal laws of its own. In the world of Spirit you need to pay close attention to the unseen. You may sense or feel in a slightly different way, but this is gradual. Sometimes this *shift* is lost among your normal activities until you feel "spaced out." At these moments it is time to reconnect with Mother Earth.

The solution to contrary Swan is:

1) Notice your surroundings and touch the Earth with your feet, hands, or both.

2) Focus on *one* reality *or* the *other*: If you are being called to visit the Dreamtime, stop what you are doing and be still. Enter the silence and empty your mind of chatter. Be receptive and open so that the message may enter your consciousness.

3) If you are just preoccupied, daydreaming, or "spacey," you need to focus on doing some physical activity. Use the reasoning side of your brain to make a list of what you need to do next, and this will stop the clutter in your mind that may be causing the confusion.

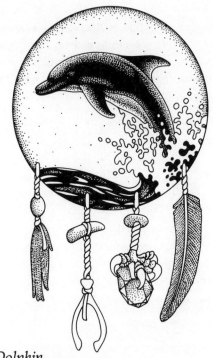

Dolphin . . .
   Breathe with me.
      Breath of the Divine,
         Manna of the Universe,
            In Oneness we entwine.

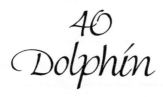

40
Dolphin

---MANNA---

Dolphin speaks to us of the breath of life, the only thing that humans cannot go without for more than a few minutes. We can live without water and food for days, but oxygen is the source of our sustenance. Within the breath we encounter the rhythm of energy that all life emits. In changing the rate or rhythmic texture of our breath, we can tap into any other life-form or creature. This is a very easy way to connect with divine energy coming from Great Spirit, as well as with your own personal rhythms.

Dolphin is the keeper of the sacred breath of life, and teaches us how to release emotions through Dolphin breath. Dolphin creates rhythm, swimming through the water and breathing before submerging, then holding its breath for the duration of underwater travel. As Dolphin comes above water again, it blows its breath out in a manner resembling the popping of a cork. We can use this same technique to pull the stopper on our tensions and create total relaxation. This is a good exercise to use before entering the silence.

Manna is life force. Manna is present in every atom, and is Great Spirit's essence. Dolphin teaches us how to use life-manna through our breath. It revitalizes each cell and organ, and breaks the limits and dimensions of physical reality so that we may enter the Dreamtime.

Dolphin was traveling the oceans one day as Grandmother Moon was weaving the patterns of the tides. Grandmother Moon asked Dolphin to learn her rhythms so that he could open his female side to her silvery light. Dolphin began to swim to the rhythm of her tide weaving, and learned to breathe in a new way. As Dolphin continued to use this new rhythm, he entered the Dreamtime. This reality was a new and different place from the seas he had known.

Dolphin came to discover underwater cities in the Dreamtime, and was given the gift of the primordial tongue. This *new language* was the *sound*-language that was brought by Spider from the Great Star Nation. Dolphin learned that all communication was pattern and rhythm, and that the new aspect of communication was sound; he carries this original pattern to this day. Dolphin returned to the ocean of the Great Mother, and was very sad until Whale came by and told Dolphin that he could return to be a messenger to the Dreamtime dwellers anytime he felt the rhythm and used the breath. Dolphin was given a new job. He became the carrier of messages of our progress. The Dreamtime dwellers were curious about the children of Earth, and wanted us to grow to be at one with Great Spirit. Dolphin was to be the link.

If Dolphin has appeared to you today, frothing through the waves in your spread, you are to be a link to some solution for the Children of Earth. This can be a time when you are to link with Great Spirit and bring answers to your own questions or to those of others. In addition, this can mean a time of communication with the rhythms of nature. You are put on notice to be mindful of your body rhythms and the patterns of energy being fed to you from the Creator. Imitate Dolphin and ride the waves of laughter, spreading joy in the world. Breathe and experience the manna so freely given. Break existing barriers and connect to the Dreamtime or Great Star Nation. Know that we are all whole in the eyes of the Everliving One.

CONTRARY:

If Dolphin appears reversed, know that you are forgetting to breathe. You may be under stress, and your body may need manna. You may be starving your cells and organs no matter how many vitamins you are taking. Your natural cycles may be fouling up. Pay close attention to your health and your feelings. If you are on edge or just tense, take time to relax and breathe the life force into your muscles. Focus on releasing old breath at the bottom of your lungs and refilling your respiratory system with regenerative manna. Breathe from the diaphragm and fill the lungs to capacity. Then exhale from the chest to the belly, allowing your body to totally relax as you breathe out.

Another message of contrary Dolphin is that many signals are carried through universal tides or waves, and you may be failing to use your sonar. To detect these wave-patterns you many need to re-align yourself with natural rhythms within your body. Then it is neccessary to use the Dolphin breath to connect to universal aware-nesses and signals.

Dolphin says to dive deeply into the water, to play by the coral reefs, and to discover the beauty of the rhythm of breath.

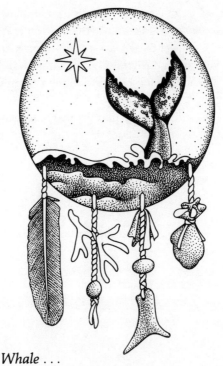

Whale . . .
        Of mighty oceans,
                You have seen it all.
                        Secrets of the ages are
                                Heard within your call.

Teach me how to hear your words,
        And how to understand,
                The very roots of history,
                        Of when our world began.

41
Whale

Whale is very much like a swimming library. Whale carries the history of Mother Earth and is said to have been placed here by the Ancients from the Dog Star, Sirius.

Biologists say that Whale is a mammal, and very possibly lived on land millions of years ago. In tribal legend, Whale's move into the ocean happened when the Earth shifted and Lemuria, the Motherland, went below the waves.

All of our petroglyphs speak of the Motherland, Mu, and the disaster that brought the red race to North America from the West, beyond the great waters. The symbols in the petroglyphs speak of the rivers and mountains crossed by our ancestors when they sought solid ground as the water receded.

Whale saw the events that led to the settling of Turtle Island (North America) and has kept the records and knowledge of the Motherland alive. It is said that Mu will rise again when the fire comes from the sky and lands in another ocean on Mother Earth. The Native medicine people are waiting for this event as the next sign of Earth changes. Earth's children will *have* to unite and honor all ways and all races in order to survive.

Whale medicine people are coded in their DNA to understand that sound frequencies can bring up records in the memories of ancient knowledge. They are usually clairaudient, or able to hear both very low and very high frequencies. They are usually also psychically developed and fairly telepathic. Many times, however, they are not awakened to their gifts until it is time to use the stored records. Many Whale medicine people are able to tap into the universal mind of Great Spirit, and have no idea how or why they know what they know. Only later, when they receive confirmation, do they begin to understand how they know or why they received the impressions.

Whale medicine teaches us to use the sounds and frequencies that balance our emotional bodies and heal our physical forms. To recall *why* the shaman's drum brings healing and peace is to align with Whale's message. The drum is the universal heartbeat and aligns all beings heart to heart.

Before the advent of speech and the primordial language, hand signs were used, and many tribes were silent most of the time. The language that was understood was the sounds of Great Spirit's other creatures, the animals.

If you pulled the Whale card, you are being asked to tap into these records and to allow yourself to be sung to by those who have the original language. We are the only creatures who do not have our own unique cry or call. Find yours. Allow your voice to use this sound to release tension or emotion. Whale signals a time of finding your origins, of seeing your overall destiny as coded in your DNA, and of finding the sounds that will release those records. You may never be the same again. After all, you are the melody of the Universe, and the harmony is the song of the other creatures. In using your voice to open your memory, you are expressing your uniqueness and your personal sound. As you open to this uniqueness, the animals that are your nine totems may then send their sounds or calls to you or through you. This will open your personal records so that you may further explore your soul's history and commune with Whale, who carries the history of us all.

CONTRARY:

If Whale has beached itself in your cards, the contrary medicine implies that you are not following your sonar or homing device. On some level you have forgotten that you hold all the answers you need to survive, to grow, and to claim the power of your chosen destiny.

It may be that you are having to deal with a lot of chatter in your head and cannot get to your personal records. If so, you may need to use other sounds to enter the silence. The drum or rattle, the Indian flute, or the sounds of nature may help. The

call of Whale is the lullaby of the tides. Rock yourself gently
and float into the world of the sea. Flow with the waters of time
and collect *your* answers — they are the only truth that will lead
to your personal pathway of knowing.

Contrary Whale is saying that you must *desire to know.* You
must seek the Whale song within you. In hearing Whale's call
you will connect to the Ancients on a cellular level, and then as
you relax into the flow of the song's rhythm you will begin to
open *your* unique library of records. It may not come all at
once. It may take practice, but if you hold the desire *to know*
close to your heart, it will be Whale's gift to you. Look to the
Great Star Nation and send gratitude to Sirius for the song
of Whale.

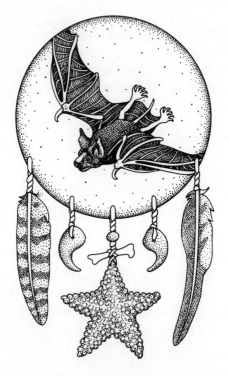

Sacred Bat . . . flew to me,
    From the darkness of the cave.
        Womb-like reflections,
            Answers it gave.
Birth, death, rebirth,
    Cycles of the whole . . .
        Never-ending,
            just eclipsed,
The journey of the soul.

42
Bat

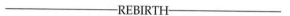
————————REBIRTH————————

Steeped in the mystery of Mesoamerican tribal ritual is the legend of Bat. Akin to the ancient Buddhist belief in reincarnation, in Central America, Bat is the symbol of rebirth. The Bat has for centuries been a treasured medicine of the Aztec, Toltec, Tolucan, and Mayan peoples.

Bat embraces the idea of shamanistic death. The ritual death of the healer is steeped in secrets and highly involved initiation rites. Shaman death is the symbolic death of the initiate to the old ways of life and personal identity. The initiation that brings the right to heal and to be called shaman is necessarily preceded by ritual death. Most of these rituals are brutally hard on the body, mind, and spirit. In light of today's standards, it can be very difficult to find a person who can take the abuse and come through it with their balance intact.

The basic idea of ancient initiations was to break down all the former notions of "self" that were held by the shaman-to-be. This could entail brutal tests of physical strength and psychic ability, and having every emotional "button" pushed hard. Taunting and spitting on the initiate was common, and taught him or her to endure the duress with humility and fortitude. The final initiation step was to be buried in the earth for one day and to be reborn without the former ego in the morning.

This ritual is very similar to the night of fear practiced by natives of Turtle Island. In this ritual, the shaman-to-be is sent to a certain location to dig his or her grave and spend the night in the womb of Mother Earth totally alone, with the mouth of the grave covered by a blanket. Darkness, and the sounds of animals prowling, quickly confronts the initiate with his or her fears.

As the darkness of the grave has its place in this ritual, so does the cave of Bat. Hanging upside-down is a symbol for learning to transpose your former self into a newborn being. This is also the position that babies assume when they enter the world from the womb of woman.

If Bat has appeared in your cards today, it symbolizes the need for a ritualistic death of some way of life that no longer suits your new growth pattern. This can mean a time of letting go of old habits, and of assuming the position in life that prepares you for rebirth, or in some cases initiation. In every case, Bat signals rebirth of some part of yourself or the death of old patterns. If you resist your destiny, it can be a long, drawn out, or painful death. The universe is always asking you to grow and become your future. To do so you must die the shaman's death.

CONTRARY:

If Bat is still hanging upside-down in the cave and immersed in darkness, you have met its contrary medicine. This position leads to stagnation of the spirit and a refusal to acknowledge your true destiny — which is always to use the talents you have to the fullest. Is there some area of your life that has dammed up and therefore stopped your desire to create? If so, look at surrendering to the death of that stagnation.

Bat can also imply that in the reversal of your natural cycle of rebirth you are trying to go at life in a backward mode. This is a breech birth, in a sense. This type of occluded understanding of how to go about freeing yourself can lead to a stillbirth if you struggle too long in the birth canal. The final outcome can be death of the body. Some people think themselves into a corner with obstacles that are illusionary. By the time they decide what to do, the opportunities are gone and old age is upon them. All of their dreams have passed them by. Reversed Bat says to use your mind, courage, and strength to insure an easy labor and quick delivery into your new state of understanding and growth. Surrender to the new life you have created from thought and desire, and bravely greet that dawn.

If you are concerned with today and tomorrow but not much further, you may forget to see further down the road. Tribal teachings say that you are responsible for future generations because you are the ancestors of the future. Whatever you do today will affect the next seven generations. Every decision, every thought, is to create a state of stagnation or rebirth for those that follow you on the Good Red Road. If you are blocking yourself, you may be blocking the generations to come.

Bat flies at night, and in the night are born your dreams. These are the dreams that build future civilizations, so nourish them well.

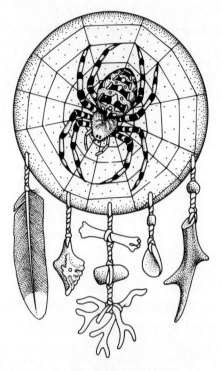

Spider . . . weaving webs of delight,
Weave me a peaceful world.
Carrying creation in your web,
Waiting to be unfurled!

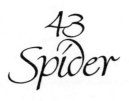
43
Spider

---WEAVING---

Spider wove the web that brought humans the first picture
of the alphabet. The letters were part of the angles of her web.

Deer asked Spider what she was weaving and why all the
lines looked like symbols. Spider replied, "Why Deer, it is time
for Earth's children to learn to make records of their progress in
their Earth Walk." Deer answered Spider, "But they already have
pictures that show through symbols the stories of their experiences." "Yes," Spider said, "But Earth's children are growing more
complex, and their future generations will need to know more.
The ones to come won't remember how to read the petroglyphs."

So it was that Spider wove the first primordial alphabet, as
she had woven the dream of the world that had become manifest.
Spider's dream of the physical world had come to fruition
millions of years before.

Spider's body is made like the number eight, consisting of
two lobe-like parts connected at the waist, and eight legs. Spider
is the symbol for the infinite possibilities of creation. Her eight
legs represent the four winds of change and the four directions
on the medicine wheel.

Spider weaves the webs of fate for those who get caught in
her web and become her dinner. This is similar to humans who
get caught in the web of illusion in the physical world, and
never see beyond the horizon into the other dimensions.

The web of fate also represents a wheel of life, which does
not include any alternatives or solutions. It is typically human
to get caught in the polarity of good or bad fortune without
realizing that we can change it at any time. If we are not decisive
enough about changing our lots in life, we may end up being
consumed by our fears and limitations.

Spider is the female energy of the creative force that weaves the beautiful designs of life. Her web has hundreds of intricate patterns which catch the morning dew.

If Spider has dropped from her web into your cards today, she may be telling you to create, create, create! Look for new alternatives to your present impasse. She can also be warning you that you are coming too close to an entangling situation. Spider could be asking you to use a journal to write out and review your progress. If you do this, you will not forget *how* you are creating a new or different phase in your life.

Spider brings a message of a different kind when she sees you becoming a bit too involved in the weaving of your life plans to notice opportunity at the outskirts of your web. If this is the case, Spider gets your attention so that you notice that something you have woven has borne fruit. Congratulations! Spider caught you just in time, before you missed the opportunity on the edge of your web *or* reality.

The most important message from Spider is that you are an infinite being who will continue to weave the patterns of life and living throughout time. Do not fail to see the expansiveness of the eternal plan.

CONTRARY:

The contrary aspect of Spider is akin to the negative side of woman. Spider will eat her mate if she gets too caught up in herself to see the validity of honoring male energy. The warrior at her side is a strong balancing force. If you have become disdainful of your mate (male or female) and have felt very superior recently, you are not honoring either your male or female side.

If you are not presently in a relationship, you may have chosen a member of your family or a workmate to harass. This type of negative criticism only breaks down relations, and is a reflection of something you hate about yourself. If you are trying to feed your ego in this manner, you have lost the game. You are entangled in the web of your own illusion about who you really are. It may be time to look at why you are being critical and why you are feeling so weak that you must attack others.

If this does not apply to your situation, take a look at another message that contrary Spider medicine brings: lack of creativity. If you fail to use your talents to get the web spinning, your lack of creativity can change into destructiveness. If you are feeling stagnant and unable to move in a positive direction, you may come to resent others who are doing well. This resentment will become a Black Widow Spider and eat you up, and the only one to mourn your demise will be you. Get moving, find joy and new ideas in the accomplishments of others, and use them to propel you into a new phase of creative spinning on your own web of delight. Observe Spider's web and find pleasure in the ideas you receive from her universal language.

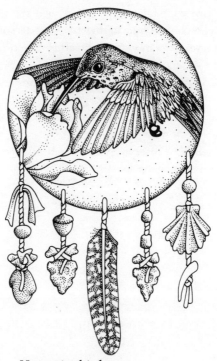

Hummingbird . . .
    Joyful little sister,
        Nectar you crave!

All the sweetness
    Of the flowers,
        Is the love you gave.

44
Hummingbird

———————JOY———————

Hummingbird is associated with the Ghost Shirt religion, which taught that a certain dance done properly would bring about the return of the animals, and that white people would disappear. Once again the Original People would know the joy of the old ways. In Mayan teachings, Hummingbird is connected to the Black Sun and the Fifth World. Hummingbird can give us the medicine to solve the riddle of the contradiction of duality.

The song of Hummingbird awakens the medicine flowers. Hummer sings a vibration of pure joy. Flowers love Hummingbird because nectar-sucking brings about the reproduction of their families. Plants flower and live because of Hummingbird.

Hummingbird can fly in any direction — up, down, backward, and forward. Hummingbird can also hover in one spot and appear to be motionless. Great Spirit created Hummingbird to be slightly different from other feathered creatures.

Because of their magical qualities, Hummingbird feathers have been used for a millennium in the making of love charms. It is said that Hummingbird conjures love as no other medicine does, and that Hummingbird feathers open the heart. Without an open and loving heart, you can never taste the nectar and pure bliss of life. To Brother and Sister Hummingbird, life is a wonderland of delight— darting from one beautiful flower to another, tasting the essences, and radiating the colors.

If Hummingbird is your personal medicine, you love life and its joys. Your presence brings joy to others. You join people together in relationships which bring out the best in them. You know instinctively where beauty abides and, near or far, you journey to your ideal. You move comfortably within a beautiful environment and help others taste the succulent nectar of life.

Hummingbird holds the Bow of Beauty which is delicately inlaid with gold and silver flowers, pearls, and precious jewels. Hummingbird disdains ugliness or harshness, and quickly flies away from discord or disharmony.

If Hummingbird has flown into your cards, get ready to laugh musically and enjoy Creator's many gifts. Drop your judgmental attitude and relax. Hummingbird will no doubt give you a flash of the spirit, darting here, there, and everywhere. Get ready for a strange new burst of energy which may send your senses reeling.

Hummingbird hears celestial music and is in harmony with it. Hummingbird may invite you to an art museum or a concert. Hummingbird energetically embraces the highest aesthetics.

Never be coarse in front of Hummingbird, for this is a fragile medicine which may have no understanding of worldly affairs. Beauty is the target, and Hummingbird's mission is to spread joy or to be destroyed. Hummingbird quickly dies if caged, caught, or imprisoned.

Follow Sister Hummingbird and you will soon be filled with paroxysms of joy, and experience a renewal of the magic of living.

CONTRARY:

If contrary Hummingbird is in your cards in any configuration, it speaks to you of matters of the heart. How or why has your heart center closed? Have you done something callous to others causing them to shut off the love they once felt for you. The contrary Hummingbird may presage sorrow and the inability to see the many blessings we two-leggeds have been given and the primordial beauty that surrounds us. If contrary Hummingbird sings its forlorn song, perhaps you should journey into your personal pain and know that your sorrow is your joy in *another* reflection.

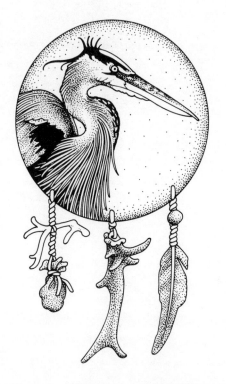

Blue Heron . . . Thank you, Sacred Waterbird,
   For sending reflections to me;
      The mirrors of the quest for life,
         The worlds that live inside of me.

Show me how relationships work,
   With my path woven within the whole.
      The lessons of kinship with all life,
         Reflecting my spirit's eternal goal.

45
Blue Heron

----------SELF-REFLECTION----------

Heron medicine is the power of knowing the self by discovering its gifts and facing its challenges. It is the ability to accept all feelings and opinions without denying any emotion or thought. Heron flies over those who are unaware of who they are and where they belong in the world. Gently dropping a blue feather to them, Heron asks that they follow their intuition and begin the empowering journey of self-realization.

If the great Blue Heron has flown into your cards today, it is urging you to dive into the watery world of feelings to seek your truth. Heron teaches you to develop your self-reflective skills so that you may come to know yourself in an intimate way. Looking at yourself through the filmy lens of self-importance, the cloudy perceptions of low self-worth, or the myopic eyes of self-pity, you will never understand your true potential or appreciate the opportunities that appear.

Heron asks that you examine yourself with a cold eye to see what you wish to improve and how you want to change. If you get stuck in the process, it may be a sign that you are being too hard or critical. Choosing to blame others and constantly pointing a finger at life's situations, instead of claiming responsibility for your actions, shows that you lack the courage to face the enemy within.

Heron medicine people are willing to look at themselves and see the truth of their motives, actions, feelings, dreams, goals, inner strengths, and inner weaknesses. In balancing those truths, Heron's medicine shows you how to meet the challenges of your personal weaknesses and how to continue developing the skills that lead to inner strength and certainty of purpose.

Are you willing to dive into the watery depths of your own feelings and discover the role of your spiritual essence? Heron is now calling you to delve deeper, to know yourself, and to trust your path. Like the Phoenix, who rises from its own ashes, Heron emerges from the unseen worlds of spirit into a new balanced sense-of-self in order to embrace its potential again and again.

The magnificence of your human spirit lies waiting for the joy of discovery, if you are courageous enough to follow the Waterbird throughout the journey. Heron reminds you that every traveler on life's journey is a messenger, and that every destination is the beginning of a new life cycle on the Medicine Wheel.

CONTRARY:

Surprise! It may be time to come up for air if Heron arrives in the contrary. Too much self-reflection can lead to self-obsession or a morbid sense of humor. If you have been looking within and criticizing yourself, watch out! It is imprudent to drown the sense of joy that usually accompanies the journey of self-discovery. You may have assumed the attitude that perfection is desirable. That may be what advertisers sell you, but that attitude leaves no room to be human. Oops! You learn some of your most valuable lessons through your mistakes. Wouldn't life be boring if everyone was a plastic clone of an ideal human?

Contrary Heron also reminds you that self-improvement is best accomplished by balancing the desire to change with gentle discernment. There are many layers of truth to understand, and wholeness is impossible to attain in one dive. You do belly flops when you become judgmental, rigid, and flat. Diving deeply into your feelings, you may emerge renewed. But, being too critical, merely floating on top of the water, you will callously break your spirit in the process. Heron reminds you to dive deeply, but do not hold your breath while waiting for instant or total enlightenment. If you do not resurface for air, the collective feelings of humanity and the infinite depth of eternity can drown you.

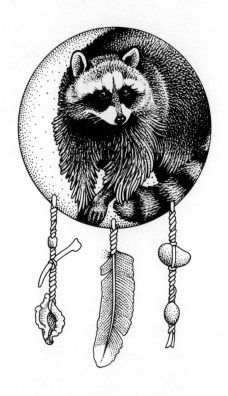

Raccoon . . . protector of the underdog,
  Provider for those who have none.
    Do you wear the bandit's mask
      To hide the good deeds that you've done?

Teach me to turn away from
  Rich rewards or worldly acclaim,
    Knowing that my generosity allows
      My warrior spirit to be reclaimed.

46
Raccoon

Raccoon carries the medicine of the protector of the underdog and provider for the young, infirm, and elderly. Often called "little bandit" by southern tribes, this Robin Hood of the animal kingdom teaches us about generosity and caring for others. When Raccoon comes your way, you are being asked to contact your inner warrior, to become a protector and generous provider for those in need. Raccoon medicine people have the uncanny ability to assist others without allowing them to become victims or dependents. Like the tribal chiefs of old, Raccoon tends to the needs of the tribe before taking anything for itself.

A troupe of Raccoons scouting for food is often a hilarious exercise in generosity. After rolling in the cornmeal or flour, they finally settle on their favorite morsels, giving the best tidbits to their lookout. Raccoons leave a watcher behind when raiding a campsite or mountain cabin, usually the dominant male. He is always fed first by the other raiders to honor his vigilance as the group's protector. This uncommon lack of greed is as rare in the world of humans as it is in the rest of the animal world. While other creatures fight one another for the best of a kill, Raccoon teaches the universal law of giving back to the source of your strength, guidance, and protection. You are also reminded that benevolence and generosity come around full circle to reward the giver.

If Raccoon wandered into your cards today, the little bandit may be telling you to look around and see who needs your strength at this time. Speak up in defense of another instead of remaining silent when others are gossiping. Maybe it is time to share the bounty of your time, energy, or possessions with the less fortunate. But remember to help those in need develop their own protector and provider skills. In all cases, Raccoon asks that you honor yourself and others equally. Provide for your own needs, or your well will be dry when you choose to give generously. Chiefs earn their Eagle feathers when they promote every human's right to self-dignity; acting in this manner brings that same honor to yourself and to your family.

CONTRARY:

If Raccoon has appeared in the reverse position, you may be robbing yourself of much needed strength at this time. Do you need an attitude adjustment? If you are wasting energy on self-pity, feeling like an underdog, do something nice for someone else. The change of focus could create more self-esteem. Observing the authentic needs in another's situation absolves self-pity. Another contrary message is denying the need to be generous or compassionate with yourself. In this case, you may not be providing enough workable options to solve your present challenges.

If you are feeling drained, it may be time to receive the gratitude of those you have helped in the past. If you have been giving too much and have forgotten to honor your own needs, Raccoon could be telling you to steal some time to be alone. The little bandit also reminds you to keep watch for "takers" who never give back. Keep yourself from feeding others who are too needy or too greedy. Balanced Raccoon medicine does not waste its generosity on those who refuse to help themselves or are too lazy to contribute or learn self-reliance.

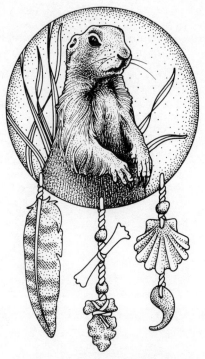

Prairie Dog . . . calls me
    when it's time to rest,

When it's time to honor
    the internal quest.

I go into retreat
    so I may see,

A way to replenish
    the potential in me.

47
Prairie Dog

---RETREAT---

Prairie Dog medicine teaches that strength and inspiration can be found by retreating into the stillness that quiets the mind. The strength of this medicine is also knowing when and how to replenish your life force. Prairie Dog medicine people tend to seek self-empowerment in silence and inactivity, where they can access dreams and visions without the intrusions of worldly chaos. When they reenter the world, they are profound and powerful anchors of calm resolve amid life's storms.

The medicine of Prairie Dog is applicable to all of the Marmot Tribe, which includes the Ground Squirrel clan, the Gopher clan, the Woodchuck clan, and the Ground Hog clan. Just as Native American warriors knew when to charge forward and when to become invisible, the Marmot tribe knows how and when to retreat. The Prairie Dog runs for the tunnels when a predator is on its trail; in the winter, it conserves energy by hibernating during the scarce time of the cold moons.

If Prairie Dog has surfaced in your cards today, it may be a warning that your body's fuel gauge is running low. You might need a day of silence or retreat from regular activities before you become too exhausted to carry on. Have you put your basic needs at the bottom of the "To Do" list? Burning the candle at both ends may weaken the punch you can normally pack when tackling the tasks at hand. Take a much needed break before you crash and burn. Prairie Dog teaches you that, in order to access gifts of inspiration and renewal, you must be at peace with yourself and rested enough to recognize the blessings being offered.

If you have been battling a situation without gaining ground, Prairie Dog reminds you that pushing too hard can create a resistance that does not allow for interaction. Take a break! Give it a rest! After a comfortable and relaxed time, you can return with a fresh perspective. In the meantime, the dynamics of the situation may have changed because your retreat allows the present challenge to work itself out. There is ample strength available if you quit pushing and go with the flow. Prairie Dog says its tunnels run both ways; now it is time to choose the backdoor exit for some rest and relaxation.

CONTRARY:

Oops! The worry bug may have bitten Prairie Dog, and it has appeared in the contrary. Has the workaholic syndrome gotten the best of your inner knowing and sensible outlook on life? Have you been tunneling in a nonproductive direction, because you forgot to come up for air, look around, and get your bearings? Have you become addicted to the adrenaline created by scurrying to catch up? If you get sick from the chaos of overactivity, you may have an unwelcome and enforced rest period at hand. Constant stress can steal your inspiration and ability to think on your feet.

Another contrary message of Prairie Dog is believing that compromise or retreat is a sign of weakness. Goodbye lie! You can get stuck in this one-way tunnel if you let your head get too big. If you cannot be still, be comfortable alone, and/or if you cannot delegate responsibility, you need a reality check. Do not be afraid to take a break, to refill your resources, and to adopt a healthy, more relaxed viewpoint. Contrary Prairie Dog also teaches that pushing too hard can have dire consequences: The cemeteries are filled with people who once believed that they were indispensable.

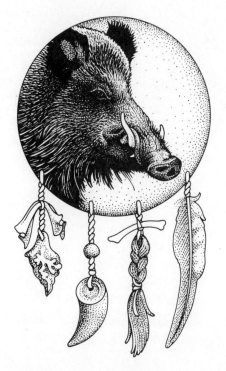

Wild Boar . . . teaches us
    to confront without fear,

Ripping apart the denials
    and lies that appear,

Testing courage, finding truth,
    its medicine will remain,

A part of every human path,
    marking the victories we attain.

48
Wild Boar

---CONFRONTATION---

Although the warrior was accustomed to the sultry heat of his bayou homeland, he was shaking as if from a cold draft. The Council of Elders had caught him telling a lie. The punishment for this offense was banishment from the tribe. To restore his honor among the People, he would have to face the Wild Boar with a knife as his only weapon. If he failed, he would die, torn apart by the ravaging tusks of the fiery-eyed beast. This prospect filled him with dread.

Then, the spirit of the Wild Boar came to him in a dream; it was enraged that the young man had broken his warrior's vows by lying. It told him that he would first have to face and conquer the self-important and deceitful beast within himself, if he hoped to survive their combat. The young warrior vowed to honor the *truth* from that moment forward; he faced the Wild Boar that day and killed the beast. The warrior kept the tusk of his adversary as a life-long reminder to always confront the weaknesses within himself.

There are several varieties of Boar, and this powerful medicine of the Warrior Clans applies to all of them. The Maya called Boar, Javelina, and the Choctaws saw the Razorback as Wild Boar. Its medicine teaches us to confront human weaknesses and to change them into strengths. The human spirit is empowered through Wild Boar's willingness to confront fears, the challenges at hand, and uncomfortable circumstances. Courageously standing tall, without running from the situations that life presents, is powerful medicine indeed.

If Wild Boar has charged into your cards today, you are being asked to confront anything or anybody that you have been avoiding. Pay attention! Embrace your warrior nature and find the courage to confront your fears. Or, are you being asked to confront a personal weakness or a career challenge? Is it time to finish a project that you abandoned thinking it might be too difficult to accomplish? Confront your feelings regarding some situation that makes you nervous or causes discomfort and bring yourself the peace of closure.

If you have been procrastinating, Wild Boar is reminding you to quit avoiding the inevitable. In all cases, it is insisting that you be fully present and mindful of what is happening and why. If you drew this card, you already possess the courage needed to confront all that life offers; just remember where you hid that courage. Challenges do not simply vanish. Unless you actively embrace your issues, you cannot reclaim your spirit's energy. Half the battle is won through the warrior's willingness to acknowledge and to accept the whole truth at all times.

CONTRARY:

If Wild Boar has appeared in the contrary position, this could be a warning: Because you have been unwilling to confront some challenge, situation, or feeling, it is about to explode in your face. It could be time to evaluate any avoidance mechanisms. Denials can vanish when you confront them with unflinching honesty. If some lie is present, now it is time to come clean with yourself or another. Have you dishonored yourself by breaking a trust? Be strong and make amends. If you do not believe that you are brave enough to confront your mistakes or denials, quit lying to yourself and acknowledge the authentic power of the honorable self within.

Remember, you can call upon Wild Boar to help cut through feelings of helplessness or weakness. Those sharp tusks can cut to the heart of the matter and reveal the valiant warrior self that you may have unwittingly abandoned.

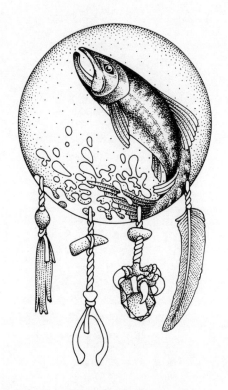

Salmon . . . keeper of inner knowing,
   Illuminate all that I can see,
      Fill me with the love of learning,
      Life's sacred wisdom offered to me.

49
Salmon

--------WISDOM/INNER-KNOWING--------

Salmon is the sacred keeper of wisdom and inner knowing who, despite strong river currents, will always return to the place of its creation. Its determination is driven by the wisdom of instinct and inner knowing, which yields a sense of purpose that cannot be thwarted by external forces. Coming full circle, Salmon medicine people finish what they begin, bringing life's events and cycles to closure.

Salmon medicine honors every encounter in life as a gathering of wisdom. It teaches that even when the flow of life seems to push you back, you can tap the hidden resources of your human spirit and personal inner knowing. The journey may not be an easy one, and the currents of public opinion may not be in your favor, but you can choose to honor the wisdom you carry and instinctually do what is right.

If Salmon swam into your cards today, it may be telling you to trust your gut feeling and inner knowing at this time. Avoid the influence of those who may have hidden agendas or who manipulate events for their personal gain. Do you need to reflect on the personal experiences that will help you decide whether the tide is ebbing, or flowing in a direction that benefits your forward movement and growth? Go back to the beginning and retrace your path to this point. The wisdom is inside you, and when honoring it, you will not go wrong.

The silver of Salmon's skin reflects many lessons. To reclaim your inner knowing, you must see the opportunity in all situations, and know that wisdom is earned through both life's easy and difficult experiences. Be willing to listen to others, as well as to the small, still voice within. Behave in a manner that honors your path. The proper use of inner knowing comes when you flow with your authentic feelings, embracing all the experiences you encounter in life as learning lessons rather than hardships. Salmon teaches you to see every bend in the river as a new adventure, with a lesson you need to learn in order to grow. That knowledge becomes authentic wisdom through applying these truths to your life.

CONTRARY:

If Salmon has floated belly-up into your cards today, recklessness may have kept you from achieving a goal. Are you ignoring the wise advice of others or your own inner voice of wisdom? Contrary Salmon may be telling you to be still for a time and find the flow again. Ask yourself where you became distracted or confused. Then imagine returning to the place you last felt certain of yourself. Feeling a sense of serenity means you are tapping your inner knowing and wisdom again.

If you have been seeking the approval of others by being a follower instead of listening to your personal knowing, it may be time to reclaim your own authority. Are you stubbornly rejecting the truth of a situation, trying to be right or in control, and overriding your instinctual wisdom or inner knowing? If so, get out of your head and get back to the wisdom found in your heart and feelings. Like Salmon, people sometimes need to backtrack upstream to see where life's meandering tributaries flowed away from the original headwaters of their certainty, wisdom, instinct, and inner knowing.

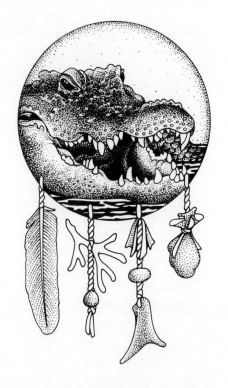

Alligator . . . Let me drop my judgments,
Accepting life with grace,
So that forlorn care and worry
Will vanish from my face.
Let me integrate each moment,
Digesting life with ease,
Counting all my experiences
As equal opportunities.

50
Alligator

---INTEGRATION---

The powerful gift of Alligator medicine is to fully appreciate
and integrate all that life offers. Gator shows us the value of thor-
oughly digesting both the pleasures and pains of life. In many
ways, Alligator's medicine is reflected in its behavior. When Gator
rolls under the water with its prey, its message is to roll with the
punches when being attacked by life's circumstances. Carefully stor-
ing its prey under a log until the meat is tender teaches us about
patience and proper timing.

Choosing to laugh when tangled in your own seriousness can
immediately diffuse the stranglehold of anger and judgments, self-
importance and inflexibility. Once your rigidity is removed, you are
free to again integrate the present set of circumstances, finding
what you may have formerly overlooked. Then you can learn
Gator's lessons on how to digest the value of any life lesson.

Gator medicine people refrain from passing judgment until
they have examined all the facts and seen all sides of any situation.
It may be time to drop opinions and judgments so that the present
situation can be fully understood. Gator might have surfaced in the
river of your life to tell you to digest the situation at hand before
making any rash moves. You could also be dealing with someone
who is too serious or rigid. If this is the case, embrace your flexibil-
ity, knowing that you are expanding beyond your former limits,
even if others are wallowing in their self-created quicksand.

Have you have been rushing through life and not taking the
time to count your victories or to digest your Rites of Passage? If
so, it could be time to honor your progress, mindful that quick-fix
solutions do not support long-term goals. Avoid getting stuck in
the duality and quagmire of the *human judgment game*. Use calm re-

solve, review your healing process and life lessons, integrating the growth you have attained.

In all cases, Gator is telling you that something may have escaped your perception. Ask yourself what viewpoint or possibility did not get factored into your assessment. Did that missing piece of the puzzle keep you from having an accurate overview of what is now occurring? If so, it is never too late to reevaluate the situation from a more integrated and flexible point-of-view. Remember, Gator's eyes and nostrils are often the only parts of its body above water while it senses its surroundings. Gator integrates all probabilities before it makes its move.

CONTRARY:

Contrary Alligator often signals a time to laugh in the face of conflict in order to survive. If Gator's belly is floating exposed on top of the water, it could mean that rash actions or thoughtless words have put you in jeopardy. Gator's treacherous jaws warn you not to fall prey to quick-fix solutions or schemes. If contrary Gator's bite has severed an artery that fed you life force, a Band-Aid will not cure your present situation. Integrate stable, long-term solutions and options.

If you have become inflexible or judgmental, detach from the muddied thinking or clouded feelings that have imprisoned your progress. In all cases, Gator reminds you to scan more than the surface, integrating all possibilities, potential risks, unexpected outcomes, and ultimate rewards. If you integrate all these viewpoints, it becomes easier to roll over and come out on top!

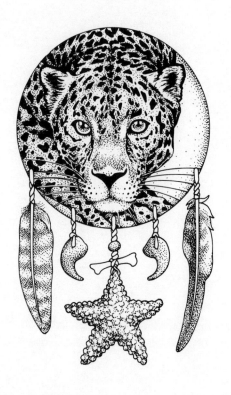

Sacred Jaguar teach me . . .
  To wear my power lightly,
    To walk with impeccability,
      To approach life with compassion,
        And to live up to the integrity of
                    my human potential.

51
Jaguar

————INTEGRITY/IMPECCABILITY————

Since the death of Skygod, the god-like being who had come from the stars and led the Maya to prosperity and a golden era of spiritual understanding, his teachings of love, integrity, impeccability, and the power of a compassionate heart had been perverted. The distortion of his Jaguar teachings had degenerated to where the priests were sacrificing human beings, foolishly cutting out the victims' hearts to reclaim the power of the golden days of the empire. Forgotten was the authentic power of the honorable and loving heart in Skygod's teachings.

The great Jaguar Spirit, who was Skygod's totem, roamed the dreams of the Maya, looking for any dishonorable behavior. Misdeeds and abuses of power had diminished the spirit of the Maya and needed to be sacrificed for the survival of the people. The priests, who had abused the authority and power bestowed on them, quaked in fear knowing that the day of reckoning had come. Jaguar brought justice by stalking their dreams and devouring their flagrantly dishonorable and greedy misdeeds.

Jaguar medicine is integrity and impeccability. Its mission is to devour the unclean aspects of human behavior. Jaguar teaches us the penalties of inappropriate behavior and offers the rewards of good medicine to those who stand in their personal integrity and walk through life in an impeccable manner.

If Jaguar is roaming your dream/reality today, its primal roar may be rewarding you for maintaining your integrity in some situation where you could have easily misused your authority. You may have been unwilling to pass judgment on another, or to be self-serving. Were you especially kind to someone or do a good deed that was unexpected? If so, allow the recognition to fill you with feelings of well-being and continue to serve with compassion and openhearted integrity.

Do not falter in your resolve to be your personal best at all times. Maintain your dignity, devotion, and compassion, holding to forthrightness and honesty, no matter what the contrary influences. Do not feed any self-important need to be an "enlightened one," treating others in a self-righteous manner. Jaguar medicine teaches you that personal integrity allows for mistakes, embraces forgiveness, and humbly makes self-directed corrections, allowing a rebalanced spirit to triumph once again.

CONTRARY:

If Jaguar is hanging upside-down from the tree limb today, you may have created an enlightenment trap for yourself. Has the misuse of authority kept you from walking your path with impeccability? Have you betrayed your personal integrity to accommodate others? Are you engaged in some activity that lessens your potential? If so, call your spirit or energy back. Integrity requires a forgiving and open heart. Compassion and mercy are also needed. Self-blame or pointing fingers at others only shows your own lack of integrity.

In the contrary, Jaguar always warns you to correct any need to control others, any abuses of influence, any form of manipulation, moralistic judgments, dishonesty, hidden agendas, envy, greed, or victim-like jealousy that may be affecting your life. If you have slipped, allowing a temporary lapse in impeccability to compromise your integrity, you need to rectify your misdeeds. Jaguar reminds us, "Become impeccable, use integrity, and you will thrive!"

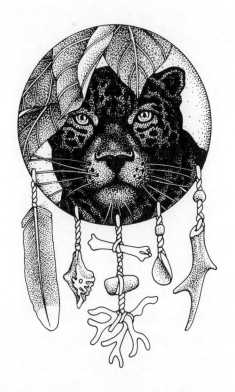

Oh Midnight Jaguar . . . Wash me with your courage.
　And steel me with your grace,
　　So I may know the value of
　　　The void of time and space.

Teach me all your lessons,
　How to face the dark unknown.
　　Then let me bravely leap
　　　Into the shadows all alone.

52
Black Panther

───────EMBRACING THE UNKNOWN───────

Black Panther slid silently through the bayou, her golden eyes catching the starlight, midnight fur soundlessly rippling over her stealthy sinew, muscle, and bone. She and her mate were the last of their kind in the homeland of the Caddo Tribe. The Panther Clan had been honored and respected by the red people of the bayou for hundreds of years. Black Panther's medicine allows human beings to face their fears and dark behaviors, exploring those internal shadowy aspects of being.

Most of Panther's tribe had been stalked and killed by the other two-leggeds, who had come across the big water and who feared their own dark natures. Those people were in need of her healing medicine. That night the Black Panther stood at the edge of the swampy bayou, sniffing at the night, trying to catch the scent of any newcomer willing to go beyond their fears and trust her medicine. No, not on this night, but she would patiently wait for one courageous explorer of the healing potential found in the dark of the unknown.

The Caddo people called her clan the Black Panther, and her tribe was known as the Midnight or Black Jaguar to the Maya. The color black is honored by the red race: Darkness is the place for seeking and finding answers, for accepting healings, and for accessing the hidden light of truth. Black Panther teaches us through our dreams to delve into the places within ourselves that need healing. She shows us how to track the unfamiliar territory found on the journey of self-discovery and to fearlessly face the unknown.

If the Black Panther has appeared today, it may be telling you not to worry about the future. Trust that you are not supposed to mentally "figure it out" at this time. You may need to confront fears of the unknown, of being less than you truly are, or an inability to simply BE. Let go of fears that appear as obstacles or barriers. Embrace the unknown and flow with the mystery that is unfolding in your life. The next step may be leaping empty-handed into the void with implicit trust. In the stillness of the void, find the will to avoid foolish interruptions, going deeper into your own self-discovery and healing process. Here you will discover Black Panther's unexpected blessings.

CONTRARY:

If Black Panther is appearing as contrary, you may be seeing situations as black or white, good or bad, with no middle ground. Be free of mental presuppositions and expectations. It could be time to do some housecleaning. Let go of negative people, limiting thoughts, or any fear of being alone. If you are out of balance, your shadow may be creating demons of fear. Enter the stillness and re-fuse to surrender your personal authority to avoidance mechanisms, justifications, or mental gymnastics. Remember, the fear of "what if" will always keep you from enjoying the present moment and life's gift is the present.

Feeling jumpy, nervous, confused, paranoid, afraid of being alone, or somehow at risk? These feelings are the shadow's domain. Tell your shadow to get lost! Then acknowledge and release any feelings of discomfort. Find the emptiness of the void and snuggle into Black Panther's midnight fur. In all cases, you are reminded that every human being emerged from the darkness of the womb; you once felt that the silence and the ebony void of this nurturing space was the safest place to BE.

Notes

_____

_____

_____

_____

_____

_____

_____

_____

_____

_____

_____

_____

_____

_____

_____

_____

_____

_____

_____

_____

_____

_____

_____

_____

_____

_____

_____

_____

_____

Notes

_____

_____

_____

_____

_____

_____

_____

_____

_____

_____

_____

_____

_____

_____

_____

_____

_____

_____

_____

_____

_____

_____

_____

_____

_____

Notes

_____

_____

_____

_____

_____

_____

_____

_____

_____

_____

_____

_____

_____

_____

_____

_____

_____

_____

_____

_____

_____

_____

_____

_____

_____

_____

_____

Notes

About the Authors

David Carson is a writer who grew up in Oklahoma. He is of Choctaw descent. He has lectured widely throughout the United States and abroad. He now lives in Sante Fe, New Mexico. His website address is *www.medicinecards.com*

Jamie Sams is an artist and writer of Cherokee, Seneca, and French descent. Her books include: *Sacred Path Cards*™, *The Sacred Path Workbook*, *Other Council Fires Were Here Before Ours* (with Twylah Nitsch), *Earth Medicine*, *The Thirteen Original Clan Mothers*, and *Dancing the Dream*. She has also written an audio adventure story with Meatball Fulton for ZBS Foundation, entitled *The Land of Enchantment*. Ms. Sams' three-tape audio distributed by Sounds True, entitled *Animal Medicine*, was voted one of the best audios of 1998 by Publishers Weekly. For futher information on her latest endeavors, her webpage is *www.jamiesams.com/nat*.

About the Artist

Angela Werneke is an illustrator and graphic designer whose artistry has appeared in numerous works that in some way serve to further healing on the Earth. Her intent is to bridge the other-than-human beings of the natural world to collective human awareness and awaken in viewers a respect and compassion for all life. Angela lives in northern New Mexico, where she nourishes a deepening relationship to place, purpose, and the next spiritual passage.